Navigating
Cancer
with the Power of
Infinity

Synergy of Science, Lifestyle
and Spirituality

ANUPKUMAR SHETTY

'A Doctor's Journey of Overcoming Cancer'

Blessings

"Infinite is the Supreme Self. This supreme self is the substratum of everything. All that which is manifest is Infinite, all that remains is Infinite.
From Infinite only Infinity can express, as Infinity is EXISTENCE. This
existence is the nature of Supreme self and this Verily is the fire of my own
being."

May this book and it's contemplation lead us to that core of our own being.

May we become the expression of pure Bliss and Peace.

Hari OM

Swami Sarveshananda, Chinmaya Mission, Dallas TX

Testimonials

"This wonderful, inspiring book is filled with important ideas and insights. These life lessons show that you have no limits to what you can do or achieve."

Brian Tracy, Author/Speaker/Consultant

"The chapters on cancer prevention are very resourceful. The chapters on yoga, meditation, plant dominant diet for holistic cancer care and prevention apply to good heart health too. I appreciate Dr. Shetty giving specific practical steps on meditation and different ways of the non-dualistic spiritual path. I recommend this cancer book to all the people who want to have good health and happiness.

Indranil Basu-Ray MD FRCP FACC, Cardiologist, Electrophysiologist, Author, Educator, and the Founder President of the American Association of Yoga and Meditation

"This book takes the reader step by step from the time of diagnosis to completion of treatment and beyond. It provides the reader with a detailed understanding of what to expect at each stage of the process. Dr. Shetty tells a rich and moving account of his journey with cancer. He talks with disarming frankness and grace and creates a distinct impression that he is sitting in the living room and talking to the reader. Dr. Shetty is also passionate about screening and encourages all eligible persons to undergo screening as appropriate. If Dr. Shetty's message of screening saves even one life, then this book has achieved its goal and Dr. Shetty's work. This is also a cancer diet book with some recipes. The book concludes with an upbeat ending with Dr. Shetty having been free of cancer for more than 15 years."

Maryada Srinivas Reddy MD, Oncologist with Baylor Scott & White, Dallas, TX

"Through his journey, Dr. Anupkumar Shetty weaves his medical knowledge with his understanding of traditional wisdom to find meaning in illness. Cancer is a difficult disease to contend with, and Dr. Shetty articulates the multi-dimensional approach needed not just for treatment, but also for pre-habilitation and rehabilitation in this holistic cancer book. During the rehabilitation period, as is often the case, Dr. Shetty faces his struggle to understand the meaning of his illness and also the meaning of life at large. Through the understanding of cancer prevention and in the deep search for the meaning of life itself, we find ourselves in Dr. Shetty's shoes leaning into existential questions and holistic cancer care: Ultimately, what is the purpose of life? And how do we free ourselves from the suffering of the physical body?"

Darshan Mehta, MD, MPH, Harvard Medical School

"Anup has used his personal story of surviving cancer to explain problem-solving, health promotion, and being unconditionally happy. A great leadership book for life and health coaches."

Sunil Tulsiani, Founder of the Private Investment Club

"I have been one of the fortunate ones to read about Dr. Shetty's account of his travails through cancer at a stage when I discovered about my own cancer diagnosis. I was already going through other health issues when this new about my diagnosis broke me mentally and I could not find an anchor to stabilize myself to fight.

I am very grateful to Dr.Shetty for giving me a copy of his holistic cancer book to read as it helped me through my journey of trying to understand my diagnosis and myself.

It is very elaborately written and for me as a reader there were many facets to it. It is not just a book about someone's life and their recovery journey, it was more about knowing him from a different perspective altogether. It is about the experiences and journey of a person who gave me hope every single day that I can survive and fulfill my dreams and ambitions.

The book is not just about a doctor's recovery from cancer - a fear that can be easily objectified and placed externally if you haven't gone through it - I was able to internalize so many of the emotions that come with the journey because I was also at the beginning of a similar experience. I definitely recommend everyone to read this book."

Anitha Udgiri, Texas USA.

"Power of Infinity is a soulful expression of experiences shared by Dr Anupkumar Shetty, my dear batchmate after undergoing a traumatic health issue. He has brought in a VIBGYOR of expressions covering medical to spiritual dimensions. Hitech medical care one side; Vedantic soulful experiences on other side. An eye opener to anyone who is in a cancer loop. His blend of spirituality with a medical issue is an unique way of handholding... To summate it's a must read cancer book and leadership book for any seeker for comprehensive solutions in life either with or without cancer. God Bless..."

Dr Bhuvaneswaran JS, Cardiologist, Director PSG Super Specialty Hospital

"The one thing that doesn't change" Proust wrote in "Remembrance of Things Past", "is that at any and every time it appears that there have been great changes."

In the course of our lives, how we deal with changes separate the men from the boys. Some rise to the occasion and dare Fate, others slip into obscurity.

Reading 'The Power of Infinity' reminded me why I admire Anup. His journey through and beyond cancer is a testimonial to the power of faith! In lieu of wallowing in self-pity and "why me" remonstrations, Anup's faith became stronger and helped him find comfort and peace and focus.

Even in the worst of times, in the face of a cancer diagnosis, he used his God-given intelligence and determination, hallmarks of his life, to guide him into a winning position. His medical training aided his recovery but his faith accelerated it.

Anup uses sports metaphors throughout his book to pass on a message to his readers. Life is a game and with courage, focus, determination and preparation, we can overcome life's challenges and become better human beings.

Clearly, humanity's battle with cancer is far from over. It is a benign illness that depending on multiple variables, can suddenly become malignant. Anup has explained this concept in simple yet profound math. Someone once said, we all have cancer cells and our responses to life's challenges acts as a trigger and turns them against our own bodies.

Anup's book is a great, unique and personal story of his journey – almost 19 years after his fight with cancer and subsequent recovery, Anup details the history of his illness and recreates "how things really were" and "what really happened."

In the 19th century, the German historian Leopold von Ranke saw it as his task to determine "how things really were," but if that could be done, it wouldn't be necessary for each generation of historians to write new books about the same subjects. We keep retelling the story of cancer and the havoc it has caused to families across the planet - partially, because new evidence is discovered, and treatments have advanced but also because with time, the way we look back at our experiences changes as the world changes.

'Navigating Cancer with Power of Infinity' is both prescriptive (a check list for fighting cancer) and inspirational – it ignites hope and reaffirms our faith in God and reminds us that we are all part of an infinite consciousness that is within us and also in everyone around us.

Mahesh Shetty CPA MBA CEO, ILE Homes

Acknowledgments

This book is the byproduct of my successful navigation of cancer. I owe that success of undoing and de-risking cancer to my 'world cup finals team' consisting of doctors, nurses, other health care providers, Methodist Dallas Medical Center, and MD Anderson Cancer Center, my wife (Mala), my children (Eesha and Krishna), my parents, my brothers (Kishore and Ashok), my sisters (Asha and Shakku), my parents-in-law, my sisters-in-law (Pramoda, Geeta, Prathima, Shammika, Sahana, Shruthi, Suparna, Riddima), my brothers-in-law (Mohan, Suresh, Ravi, Shashi, Sanskrit, and Sai), my co-brothers (Vinod, Ravi, Shrinath, Chetan, Vicky and Dasharath), my co-sisters (Akshata, Ashwita, Vaishnavi, and Aishwarya), my uncles (Sundar, Vasanth, and Sugandh), my aunts, my cousins, my nephews, my nieces, my friends, my religious guides (Swami Sarveshananda from Chinmaya Mission, Swami Bodhananda of Sambodh Foundation, and my friend, Dr Raju), my mentor (Late Dr. Dimitrios George Oreopoulos), my colleagues at Dallas Nephrology Associates, many family members, and friends.

Thanks to my friend and oncologist, Maryada Srinivas Reddy, who was the first person that I asked for help. He played a very pivotal role in providing all the medical information and guiding me and my family through all that I have gone through right from the beginning. Dr. (Late)

Karl Brinker from Dallas Nephrology Associates helped me make some crucial decisions in the beginning and I thank him for that.

I thank, Dr. Cox, who was my treating oncologist in Dallas, an epitome of knowledge, humility, and compassion. Thank you for working with the doctors at MD Anderson, providing me the best care that I got even though it was unconventional at that time, involving me in my care and most importantly, saving me. You had the humility to be open to suggestions from doctors at MD Anderson Cancer Center and the wisdom to personalize the regimen to me. Thanks to Vanessa, my chemotherapy nurse at Texas Oncology in Dallas, for being very compassionate and knowledgeable.

My oncologist at MD Anderson, Dr. Ajani was indeed a divine incarnate for me. He was kind enough to call me even before seeing me for the very first time. He was going to travel abroad the following week, but he gave me his cell phone number so I could call him if needed over the weekend before he would fly out on the following Monday. Even though I did not call him during that weekend it was very reassuring to know that he was willing to take my call despite not knowing me till then. Dr. Ajani was the Chief of Gastrointestinal Oncology at MD Anderson Cancer Center at that time. Thanks to Nemiraj Rai, my good friend who introduced me to Dr. Ajani.

Thanks to Dr. John Skibber, a very skilled and world-renowned surgeon at MD Anderson Cancer Center who specializes in operating on colon and rectal cancers. He specializes in preserving the anal sphincter in people with rectal cancer so colostomy can be avoided. He did exactly that to me. Thanks to the anesthesiologists who made my surgery painless and minimized pain during my recovery (it is impossible to make recovery entirely painless!) at MD Anderson Cancer Center (MDACC). Dr. Skibber's nurse practitioner at that time was very helpful in getting me in to see Dr.

Skibber within two weeks of diagnosis. Later during the course of my care, Dr. Skibber had a different nurse practitioner, Elizabeth Wolf who used to see me during follow-up. Elizabeth was the epitome of compassion and love. I thank both of them for being special in their own ways.

Thanks to Dr. Armond Schwartz, the gastroenterologist at Methodist Dallas Medical Center for making the initial diagnosis and for being available for my ups and downs since then; Dr. Narinder Monga, a very skilled colorectal surgeon at Methodist Dallas for guiding me well soon after the diagnosis and since then; Dr. Slomovich, the radiation oncologist at Methodist Dallas for prescribing me the right dose of radiation with precision and his radiation technicians; Misty, for providing me warm towels during radiation therapy at Methodist Dallas; all the nurses, social workers, patient care technicians, physical therapists, respiratory therapists, dieticians and other health providers at MDACC and Methodist Dallas Medical Center (MDMC); the radiologists and pathologists at both MDACC and MDMC for their behind the door contributions to my recovery.

Of course, my regular pals in random order: Sumit and Purnima, Seema, Sudipta, Sujata and Ramki, Dhruv and Savita, Kalvala and Geeta, Vijji and Raj, Manju and Vivek, Kanan and Vinay, and Ganesh and Anita have been constant pillars of unconditional support for me and my family, I owe them myself. They are the 'constants' in my life. I became closer to them over the years. Gopal and Anand have always been there for me, thanks to them. Thanks to Sangita and Ram, Mahesh and Sandhya, Gunapal, Sudha, Arti, Raymon, and many others who have helped me in various unique ways.

Thanks to Late Dr. Shyamala Nair (Shyamala Aunty), my 'mother' in America, an epitome of love and infinite spiritual knowledge that she shared with people in the community for over 40 years before she passed on. My thanks to Sriram Sarvotham, Ph.D., a very good friend, a great teacher for teaching me about yoga and its connection to spirituality and real life. He is extremely knowledgeable and has the brilliant skill of communicating it in a simple way. I know many family members, colleagues, and friends have cried and prayed for me; they still do when I get stomach upset for any reason. If I mention all their names, it will cover several more pages and it would still be an incomplete list. I thank them all every day and every moment of my life.

My colleagues in Dallas Nephrology Associates (DNA) have been extremely supportive. Dr. Velez, who was the president of Dallas Nephrology Associates at that time, made it a point to come to Houston on the day of my surgery to see me. He comforted my family members and reminded them that he was part of my family. One of my DNA colleagues, Dr. (Late) Freda Levy used to call me every day to check on me after surgery and assigned that responsibility to another colleague if she were to go somewhere out of town. They never asked me when I was going to be back at work. Samina, I remember your voicemail. I am here because of all these team members who played different roles in my game of world cup finals of fighting cancer.

Finally, I thank God, 'the Infinity' for healing me. The older I get, the more randomness I see in this world, and I believe that there is a force that drives us wherever we are driven to. You can call that force by whatever name you want. My force drove me to wherever I am today. I am grateful to that force. God, Brahman, 'Now', 'One', the 'Infinity' that I reside in, right now and every time and everywhere and keeps me going, enlightens me, heals me, strengthens me and keeps me alive, keeps me going, keeps me growing, and keeps me glowing! Please join me undo cancer!

Dedication

I dedicate this work to my brother, Kishore, whose body left this earth on February 5, 2018, after a brief illness. He crafted my life. He epitomized love, joy, humility, and hard work. I owe him everything that I am today. Kishore (I called him 'Mallanna', which means 'big brother' in my native language, Tulu) left for Mumbai at the age of 12 from our village in rural India when he started working without missing school. Child labor was probably not illegal in those days. As he grew, he took full responsibility for his siblings' education without any compromise and his parents' wellbeing. He always offered help even when he was heaped on loan. He knew to give even when he did not have much. He was always willing to help people. He was a very active leader in the hotel owner's community in New Bombay and eventually became the President of the Hotel Owners' Association.

He was also an ardent devotee of the Hindu deity Ayyappa Swamy. He visited the Ayyappa Temple in the southern state of Kerala once a year, every year for over 18 years, and took many devotees there, including me, to the shrine. He helped build the Ayyappa temple in New Bombay in India. He went to the extent of leveraging his own primary house for the temple loan. I thank Mr. Suresh Shetty, a community leader and the president of that temple in Nerul, Navi Mumbai for releasing my sister-in-law from this liability in 2021. My brother merged with God at the age of 61 years after a brief illness. I miss him dearly every day of my life. His was a short life that will live in many hearts forever. I can easily write an inspiring book on him if I have to write everything about him. Thank you 'Mallanna' for crafting my life.

I also dedicate this work to my parents. My father, Late Mr. Neere Konkebail Mahabala Shetty, instilled uncompromising values of being truthful in my life, and my mother (Late Mrs. Mundkur Doddamane Sushila Shetty) sowed the seed of tireless hard work at a very young age in me. My father was a simple man. He was a farmer. His main contribution to my life is his zero tolerance for lying. He instilled that value in my life at an early age, and I have tried to follow it to a large extent. His other quality was that he did not take much risk in his life. He never gambled and never allowed us to gamble, even for fun, including playing cards. Most of his children did not take up that quality of his. All of his children ended up becoming educated risk-takers and that has served us well. I think my mother has impacted my life much more. She is my tireless hero. She worked hard all her life and refused to slow down till she passed in 2021 at the age of 88. We, her children, had to beg her to slow down and justify why it is alright to slow down. She taught me to be accountable for my life. Act, you must! We are all destined to be doers. We must act and do our duties as a service to an infinitely stronger power that is our power and light. Results will follow as the byproduct of our actions without seeking them, without claiming our right on them.

I must remember and dedicate my work to my grandmother, Late Mrs. Meenakshi Dasu Shetty. I spent a lot of my childhood life with her and she was the epitome of love. She was the epitome of giving even when she did not have much to give. She was very creative in giving without expecting anything in return. She was a perfect example of how an illiterate person can be very educated. I hope to emulate her. I never grew up going to Sunday schools like Chinmaya Mission. But she was a living example of 'give more than what you take', which I learned formally at Chinmaya Mission later in my life in the USA. My brother, Kishore, is a nice amalgamation of my grandmother, mother, and father. He got the best of all of them! My humble gratitude and salutations to my big brother, Mallanna.

Contents

SECTION 1: GLIMPSE OF THE BOOK

Foreword I: He Left No Stone Unturned!

This is a fascinating story of a cancer survivor—how he coped with it when the news was broken to his unbelieving ears, upending his charming world of a successful and fulfilling professional and family life, the agony of mentally preparing himself and close family members for a seemingly never-ending painful journey of radiation and chemotherapy followed by a possibly life-threatening surgery, the discomforts of incontinence, the eerie feeling of a pouch filled with one's feces hanging from the belly, long sleepless nights of creepy thoughts, and the subsequent triumph in the 'world cup final'. Himself being a nephrologist, Dr. Shetty saw it all coming like an avalanche, which was scarier than the real one. Sometimes we feel that in such cases ignorance is blissful. Experience of intense and prolonged pain teaches you valuable life lessons. The scientific, rational mind of this practicing doctor desperately searched for the meaning of pain and suffering in the internet, philosophical books, spiritual talks, religious works, in temples, mosques, churches, and synagogues. He left no stone unturned, roaming from pillar to post, finally finding his secure harbor in the non-dualistic vision of oneness, a place where no cancer, for that matter, no disease can ever enter: our true home—the Infinity, Brahman, hidden in each one's heart. Dr. Shetty is a tough guy, in his own quiet way, soft-spoken, pleasant and ever-smiling, kind and hardworking, brilliant, and possessing a unique knack with words that captures his inner thoughts and feelings graphically. His humor shines through even when he explains wrenching pain. His sad smile has a way of communicating his eternal and indefatigable faith in himself and God. He seems made of diamond, unflinching in his resolve to beat cancer, by befriending and then befooling it. The only time a trace of anger flashed in his mind was when a thoughtless evangelist tried to proselytize in the pretext of saving him at his most vulnerable moment. But that anger was only an expression of his self-respect and self-rootedness. When I closed the book with a sense of having traversed through eternity, tears of aching joy welled up in my half-closed eyes. I realized that it takes an ecosystem of faith, family, and friends for true healing, which is nothing but a transcendental experience of having come home.

SWAMI BODHANANDA SARASVATI

Chairman, Sambodh Foundation INDIA &

The Sambodh Society Inc. USA

Author of "Inclusive Leadership: Perspectives from Tradition and moder-

nity"

Foreward II: Conquering Cancer and Enjoining the Infinity!

Anup is a dear friend, a great physician, and a lovely person. He is a very good storyteller. You just have to listen to him when he speaks and read what he writes. This book is like a calming brook with pure waters of action and devotion flowing between the banks of medical knowledge and Vedic wisdom.

There is so much known about cancer. And yet, there is still much more to know about its prevention, management, and recovery. Anup's ability to explain all the cutting-edge medical knowledge is very impressive. The intricacies explained in a simplified language for the benefit of non-medical people are very impressive. His illustrations and explanations of the preparation for diagnostic processes and daily enemas are very useful.

This is his own journey of life from cancer to cure, hateful disease to a state of love and ease, uncertainty to Infinity, fear to fearlessness, apprehension to achievement, and from doubtful human traits to divine genuine personality. It's our own story with or without cancer.

Anup narrates his childhood and adolescence, his life before and after the experience of cancer in a simple style with many profound messages. He explains the microcosmic nature of the body as nothing but a part of the macrocosm, emphasizing the importance of maintaining harmony with five great elements to make our body a sanctum sanctorum. His simplicity amid complexities and his unflinching faith and steadfastness in tough times will inspire us and make us better, stronger, and healthier human beings.

The real cancer is in us. It is our ignorance, lack of awareness of the "self" and the relentless sorrow. We only are responsible for making our world and life more miserable and more cancerous. The misery is born within us, grows silently, and spreads rapidly to destroy us. The insatiable desire, uncontrollable anger, and unending greed is a dreadful triad. This triad of desire, anger, and greed in us is primarily the cause of pain and suffering along with another triad of overpowering delusion, unwanted pride, and overwhelming jealousy. This sixfold enemy is as dangerous and as cancerous.

Anup gives us the solution to fight and win over these opponents with love, happiness, and grace, taking the help from Bhagavad Gita, Patanjali Yoga Sutras, Buddhist views, Adi Shankara's hymns, Ramana Maharshi's teachings, and his personal experience with great saints and swamis.

Seeing divinity everywhere, in everyone, and everything is explained through his own experience of reading, singing, writing, and practicing. He quotes Upanishads and the most profound Vedic sayings such as *'Tat Tvam Asi'* aptly with lucid explanations and refers to some of the contemporary books and personalities also.

Each of us has our own faith and we choose to take a path that suits us. We follow it with respect and reverence. He tells us firmly to respect others also equally well, for their own views and faith. We may have our own version of a religion or spiritual practice but it should not lead to conversion by imposing one's own views on others. We can converse but not convert.

He goes through more than 50 years of his life in this book of biography (if I may call it so), giving tips to prevent cancer for a life that is healthier and happier. He infuses the power to face the pain and painful situations in our life. He invokes the innate divinity and awakens the spirituality in us with guidance not just from the texts but through what he himself experimented and experienced.

He faced the mighty cancer, treating not as an enemy but as a respectful opponent with utmost self-confidence and faith in Almighty. He invoked his innate strength and drew even more strength from the supreme consciousness. He played the most important game of his life with precision, taking the right decisions at each given time, always maintaining equipoise with an attitude of gratitude to finally win the game like a true champion.

Aum Tat Sat

Weal be to All!

N V Raju, MD FRCP

Neonatologist, Author

Preface

'You have within you, right now, deep reserves of potential and ability that, properly harnessed and channeled, will enable you to accomplish extraordinary things with your life. The only real limits on what you can do, have, or be are self-imposed. They do not exist outside of you.'

Brian Tracy

According to the American Cancer Society, one in two men and one in three women in the US will have cancer at some point in their lives. In addition, cancer has replaced heart disease as the number one killer of Americans under the age of 85. The World Health Organization determined cancer is the second leading cause of death globally, accounting for an estimated 9.6 million deaths, or one in six deaths, in 2018. According to American Institute of Cancer Research nearly half of US cancers can be prevented by changing our daily habits. The cancer burden can also be reduced through early detection of cancer and management of patients who develop cancer. Prevention also offers the most cost-effective long-term strategy for the control of cancer. Those who don't ever manifest cancer end up doing so because their immune system and lifestyle have managed to prevent cancer. Those who have survived cancer and not developed recurrence of that cancer and have not developed another cancer have been successful in surviving and preventing cancer. Those who survive and prevent more cancers have to liberate themselves from cancer. This is a mental and spiritual process. I have survived cancer of the terminal part of the colon, also called the rectum, and I want to share my story of how I survived it. I also want to share how I prevented cancers after getting one and have liberated myself from cancer. There are many books written on surviving and preventing cancer. I have not come across any books covering surviving, preventing, and liberating from cancer. I have read some of them and believe that everyone has a unique story; all these stories are different and inspiring. I have mine, which may be a little different, a little bit unique, a little bit sweeter, a little bit bitter, a little bit saltier, a little bit spiritual, maybe a little bit like yours, and maybe a little bit not like yours. Every story is worth sharing. According to Charles Darwin, no two individuals are similar. Indeed, no two journeys are similar in life. But I know that I am more like you than I am not, no matter who you are, no matter which part of the world you are in, no matter whether you have had cancer or not. My story may be like yours because I live in the United States. It may be like yours because I was born in India. It may be like yours because I am a father, a brother, a son, a son-in-law, a brother-in-law, a co-brother, a friend, a scientist, a physician, or simply a human being. It may be like yours because I have not eaten much animal-based food in my life. It may be like your story because I was only 41 years of age when I was diagnosed with cancer, a little bit earlier than the usual age of presentation of colorectal cancer. I had no family history of cancer. The various other reasons why I may be like you is because I had cancer; I had spent 30 years of my life in India and eleven years in North America at the time of my diagnosis of cancer. There are infinite ways why I am like you and infinite other ways I am not. I hope my story will resonate with many of you for good reasons and help heal and deal with cancer better. If you are a caregiver, I hope that this book will guide you to help a family member or a friend dealing with cancer. If you are suffering from cancer, the book will inspire and fill you with the courage to conquer it by following certain methods, adopting a certain lifestyle, and unveiling the infinite power within you. The book is also a resource for understanding the factors that cause cancer and may hopefully help you prevent cancer.

I first realized that I owed myself and my family the best effort to get the best available care on this whole earth. I simply felt that I owed my family to get better. I also felt that the best effort had to come together the first time ever. I felt fortunate and grateful to be in a place where the best treatment was accessible to me. I felt fortunate and blessed that the USA has some of the finest cancer centers in the world. I also felt grateful that I had health insurance and other resources to afford the necessary care, even though I grew up with very limited resources. I felt grateful that I had an amazing group of family and friends I would never trade for anything else. I felt grateful that I learned about the 'Infinity' within me that gave me infinite strength to heal myself.

This book focuses initially on 'survival' by building the finest team, coming up with the best plan, and executing the best plan. Many chapters describe various logistics of cancer care. Most chapters are not unique to colorectal cancer and hence will benefit people with any kind of cancer and anyone whose family is affected by cancer. If you want to help anyone with cancer, this book is for you. In fact, the book is, in many ways, about problem-solving and hence will benefit all the world's problem solvers, including all of us. Some very important leadership lessons here can benefit management students.

The second part of the book focuses on the prevention of cancer. Prevention includes prevention of recurrence of cancer and prevention of another cancer since having one cancer does not build immunity against other cancers. In fact, having cancer once and having chemotherapy and radiation increases the risk of developing new cancer. This book may also inspire health coaches, life coaches, and students of 'healthy living' because it is all about good values, setting goals, coming up with an action plan, and executing it. There is a reference to some very important teachings from the scriptures. In many ways, these universal teachings apply to all of us irrespective of our faith. I am introducing the concept of 'liberation' from cancer and experiencing 'Infinity.' Liberation is somewhat a mental and spiritual process. One gets liberated by the power of knowledge. Knowledge involves the knowledge of the science of genesis and the end of cancer. At a spiritual level, liberation involves the knowledge that what is permanent is only true and what is impermanent is untrue. I do not want to overstate the experience of Infinity. I am not stating that I am an enlightened person. I know that I am not. In some ways, I am stating that 'experiencing Infinity' does not have to be the exclusive property of a small number of extremely spiritually evolved prophets, saints, and masters. In some ways, I am democratizing God by stating that God belongs to everyone to experience in this life. Since my body and the cancer affecting the body are impermanent, it becomes untrue. The real 'I' will always be 'I' and hence true. The realization that I am not this body or mind is liberation.

Knowing this, cancer is a transient experience and hence is not the real truth, even though the experience of having cancer is valid and real at the time of having it. By stating that cancer is a transient experience, I am not suggesting that you should not take care of it. In fact, you should make sure that it will be a transient experience. I would go to the extent that you should try to eliminate cancer as though there is no tomorrow. You should try to eliminate cancer as though it is the last game of your life. I did exactly that and that is the reason my wife has a husband today and my children who are now adults have a father. I am hoping that this book will play a role in healing yourself or your loved one. I am hoping that this will help you survive cancer and possibly write a story of your own and publish it! I am hoping that this book will help you become a better problem solver. I am hoping that this book will help you become a better leader. I am hoping that this will help you prevent cancer. I am hoping that this book will help you find and experience the divine infinite strength in you. I hope this book will help you experience Infinity within you, right here in this life, right now, without having to wait to die to experience that heaven which is a mystery. I am not denying the presence of heaven that you may be hoping to go to after death. I am just confessing that I do not know if heaven exists and there are many like me in this world who do not know if there is heaven.

My existence is unquestionable. My experience of my body is unquestionable. Remember, 'you' experience 'your body' just like I experience my body. I am the 'experiencer' of 'my body.' Can 'the experiencer (I)' be the same as 'the object or subject of experience (my body)?' Can 'the experiencer' and 'the subject that is experienced' be the same? The general wisdom is that they cannot be the same, just like the pen in my hand cannot be me. That means, 'I', the experiencer, is different from 'my body', the subject/object being experienced. I hope you will realize the infinitely powerful Infinity within you, that is divine, fearless, enemy-less, birthless, deathless, self-effulgent, eternally true, and infinitely conscious, right now, right here. That 'Infinity' is 'the experiencer' in you that witnesses the changes that your body and mind go through. I would like you to unleash and unveil that 'Infinity'.

Even though survival, prevention, and liberation are interdependent, the focus is different in different stages. 'Survival' focuses on the 'act' of getting rid of cancer, in other words, it is focused on strategic 'action' (karma) of getting optimally treated. 'Prevention' involves understanding the biology of the genesis of cancer and taking measures to prevent the genesis of cancer. 'Liberation' involves the path of 'knowledge' about 'Who Am I?'. It is somewhat a spiritual process of experiencing the Infinity that is part of each living entity in this universe including 'I' in me, but it also involves knowing the science of spirituality and keeping spirituality relevant to getting rid of and preventing cancer.

Being a doctor, I see myself as a scientist and think of everything from the lens of a scientist. But being a spiritual human being, I also see many things and for that matter, everything in life, from a spiritual lens as well. I go back and forth between validating spiritual teachings from scientific evidence and scientific happenings from spiritual teachings. Most of the spiritual teachings that I have studied are from Ancient Eastern Hindu texts such as Upanishads and Bhagavad Gita. I have studied different Hindu philosophies like yoga (self-awareness by practicing eight limbs of yoga through the discipline of body and mind), dualism (and the individual souls exist as independent realities, and these are distinct), qualified non-dualism (ultimate reality [] and the human soul are different but with the potential to be identical), and non-dualism (ultimate reality)] and the human soul are identical and all reality is interconnected oneness). These are interdependent philosophies and I personally have gone back and forth between these at different times in my life.

A large portion of Hindus and all the western religions such as Christianity, Judaism, and Islam believe in dualism where a person is devoted to and in love with an almighty God, and the devotees request and pray for healing and betterment of life. This is purely based on 'faith' that the almighty God exists and surrendering to that almighty God. The advantage of this approach is that it is conventional and heavily institutionalized and hence is readily available. There isn't much prerequisite to this practice except for 'faith' in God and 'love' towards God. The disadvantage is that it can be questioned by science and intellect since it is based on firm faith that there is God. In this philosophy, God, if exists, is an afterlife experience and hence one has to die to experience God or heaven and is not available in this life. That God is 'up there!'. That means that God is not here for me because he is 'up there'. When someone dies, we say that he or she is in a better place with 'the man up there'. But how do we know that God is a 'man'? And how do we know that God is 'up there, how far up is 'up there', and where is 'up there'? There is always a question, 'if God exists, why is he/she not here for me when I need him/her the most?' If God does not exist, you only get to live with the hope that God is up somewhere!

Yoga and some sects of Hinduism, Buddhism, Sikhism, and Jainism are based on self-inquiry and based on the experience of the divine or the 'nothingness (*shoonya*)' or '*NirvaaNa*' within the self. The advantage is that 'self' is a fact and cannot be questioned. It is experiential, hence is available today, and cannot be questioned if one experiences it. The only problem is that not many people might experience it. Hence the non-experiencer still has to live with the hope that someday he/she will experience 'it'. Non-duality, a large part of Hinduism, is an experience of 'infinite consciousness is Brahman/God', 'you are that divine reality', or 'I am that divine reality.' It has shades of duality with devotion, love, and faith leading to self-inquiry and self-experience, further leading to the knowledge and experience of 'I am the divine reality', and 'I am part of infinite consciousness, Brahman.' This is also experiential and is available in this life, right now, to all of us. One does not have to wait to die and have an after-life experience of visiting heaven. Hence, once you get the firm knowledge of the infinite consciousness within you, you have it and it cannot be questioned. It is less experience-based and more knowledge-based and hence is available to those who are open to acquiring this knowledge.

I have been heavily benefited from believing in the non-dualism philosophy to the core with full honesty to myself. I think non-dual philosophy has helped me solve problems, deal with pain, find the best healers and heal myself by finding infinite strength in myself and coming across people with infinite knowledge and potential. A detailed discussion of these different philosophies is beyond the scope of this book. But to put it easy, non-duality is the knowledge that real 'I' is an inseparable part of the 'Infinite Consciousness' who is addressed as Brahman or God or Infinity just like how a wave is inseparable from the ocean, clay is inseparable from the clay pot and gold is inseparable from the golden necklace. It is as true as the water molecule in the wave or the ocean and as true as the unchanging truth of the clay pot is made entirely of clay. While the pot can change shapes and forms, clay will always be clay. It is as true as the gold in the ornaments, no matter what shape it takes. I have admitted to this belief unapologetically throughout the book and in my real life. This knowledge has helped 'liberate' myself from cancer.

'Unleash the power within'

-Tony Robbins

If you think of it, all of us will find ourselves in different shades of 'non-dualism' in different phases of life irrespective of which religion one belongs to. This is especially true in our quest of seeking excellence in life. We see this in people who are unveiling excellence in their lives. We see this in people who profess excellence. We see different shades of 'non-duality' in the teachings of legendary business leaders, legendary coaches like Phil Jackson, and legends in different fields of life. The teachings like, 'unleash the power within' by Tony Robbins, 'go and express yourself', 'do your best', 'go and enjoy the game', 'be yourself', 'power of now' (of Eckhart Tolle fame), 'power of ONE', 'Ik Onkar', 'Inner Engineering' are all different shades of 'non-duality' written thousands of years ago in the Upanishads, the ancient Eastern Hindu texts.

"If there is God, I must see God!"

"Religion is not a matter of belief, it is a matter of experience."

-Swami Vivekananda

To put it very simply, survival is the path of action (Karma) and prevention is the path of faith with knowledge, and liberation from cancer is the path of knowledge with faith culminating in the experience of 'Infinity.' But there is a lot of overlap in these processes and about 'how' and 'when' of these processes. Prevention is part of survival, liberation is part of prevention, and both prevention and liberation are parts of survival.

I have a few suggestions for you, the reader, about how to read this book. Ideally, I would love for you to read the whole book and understand everything that is packed in it. But you may be able to skip a few pages and even some chapters depending on your interests and background. The chapter on the description of mathematical ways of explaining the genesis of cancer may be only for mathematically inclined readers. The chapter on the specific practice of meditation was meant to be specific to help those who want to try to meditate. Some parts of the section on experiencing 'Infinity' by a commoner have some words in the Sanskrit language, but you will be able to understand the contents without trying to understand the verses in Sanskrit.

I have added some new information in this edition of my "Power of Infinity" series and modified the title to direct the book to those affected by cancer, either by having cancer, wanting to help somebody with cancer, or wanting to help people prevent cancer.

I wish you blissful reading, a blissful experience, and a joyful cancer-free life. It would mean a lot to me if you could please leave an honest review now at www.amazon.com or the Amazon website of your country to help more people.

Anupkumar Shetty

Introduction

My three steps to deal with cancer:

- **Survive cancer: Play like it's the last game of your life**

- **Prevent cancer: Harmonize the five elements of the microcosm (You) and the macrocosm (the Universe), incorporating American Institute of Cancer Research guidelines and the pillars of Lifestyle medicine, creating a synergy of science, lifestyle, positive psychology and spirituality**

- **Experience Infinity: You are divine and have infinite strength and infinite power. Unveil it!**

I am a 2004 batch of survivors from cancer of the terminal part of the colon, also called the rectum. As you might know, cancer is the leading cause of death in the United States now and an important cause of death elsewhere in the world as well. As we conquer infections and malnutrition, cancer and other non-infectious medical problems are becoming more important causes of illness and death all over the world. At the age of 41 years with a young family consisting of my wife, two children aged 6 and 10 years, and multiple family members and friends, it was an unpleasant experience for me, to put it gently. I owe the victory in dealing with cancer to very skilled doctors, scientists, nurses, and other healthcare providers, my supportive family and friends, and most importantly, God who empowered me, enlightened me, energized me, blessed me, healed me, and merged with me.

The is part of the digestive system in the body. The digestive system absorbs and assimilates the nutrients like vitamins, minerals, carbohydrates, fats, proteins and water from foods and helps pass waste material out of the body. The colon is the first part of the large intestine and is about five feet long. Together, the rectum and anal canal make up the terminal six to eight inches of the large intestine. The anal canal ends at the anus. The rectum's primary function is to store formed stool in preparation for exiting the body. The inner lining of the rectum is more like that of the colon and hence cancers of the colon and rectum are often described as colorectal cancers. The treatment approach including the choice of chemotherapy drugs is similar except that the sequence of treatment options is different due to the anatomical differences of the colon and rectum. The inner lining of the anus is more like the skin and the draining lymph nodes are different. Hence the treatment of anal cancer is very different from the treatment of colorectal cancers. Colorectal cancers tend to be more responsive to chemotherapy than anal cancers.

There are three important layers of the rectum: from inside to outside, these layers are the innermost mucosal layer, then the muscular layer, and the outer serosal layer. Most of the rectum does not have a serosal layer and is surrounded by 'filling tissue' called connective tissue. The lack of serosa makes management of rectal cancer different from cancer affecting the rest of the colon. Lymph nodes are part of the immune system and assist in protection from harmful materials (including , bacteria, and cancer cells) that may be threatening the body by acting as the gatekeepers. Lymph nodes surround every organ in the body, including the rectum.

Cancer cells can spread locally, from the rectum to the lymph nodes on their way to other parts of the body or distant organs such as the liver, lungs, and other organs via the bloodstream. Spread by bloodstream is usually rare except in more advanced diseases. Like colon cancer, the prognosis (odds of recovery) and treatment of rectal cancer depends on the extent of the spread of cancer to the rectal wall, surrounding lymph nodes, distant lymph nodes, and remote organs. Treatment involves radiation, chemotherapy, immunotherapy and surgery in different combinations and different sequences depending upon the extent of the disease and goals of treatment. As far as possible the goal of treatment is to be cancer-free, but in advanced stages or advanced age, the goal can be more palliative. This is especially true if the risks and side effects of treatment are felt to be worse than the disease particularly in those with limited expected life expectancy.

Colo-rectal cancers develop usually over years. The actual cause is not known, but risk factors include increasing age (over 50), smoking, excessive alcohol intake, family history, high-fat intake, obesity, or a family history of polyps or colorectal cancer or inflammatory bowel disease.

The common symptoms of rectal cancer include a change in bowel movements including diarrhea, constipation, alternating diarrhea and constipation, a sense of incomplete evacuation of the rectum or bleeding from the rectum; other symptoms include fatigue, shortness of breath, dizziness, and/or a fast heartbeat, small diameter stools, abdominal discomfort like pain, bloating, fullness, cramps, and weight loss.

For diagnosis and further evaluation, examinations and tests include fecal occult blood testing, digital rectal examination, and colonoscopy* and biopsy of the lesion, CT//PET imaging studies along with routine blood tests, and detection of carcinoembryonic antigen (CEA). The ultimate diagnostic test is biopsy and further testing of the tissue. In addition to the microscopic examination of the tissue, sophisticated genetic testing of the tissue guides target-oriented chemotherapy and immunotherapy.

Colonoscopy is a procedure to look inside the rectum and the colon for polyps (small pieces of bulging tissue), areas, or cancer. A colonoscope is a thin, tube-like fiberoptic instrument with a light and a lens for viewing. It also has a tool to remove polyps or tissue samples and to stop bleeding. The tissue obtained is then checked under a microscope and subjected to more sophisticated testing that takes a few days.

What Healed Me and How?

"Whoever has the four qualities of courage, vision, intellect, and skill, such a person will not fail in any task."

Valmiki Ramayana: Sundarakanda verse 198

I recovered because I got the best chemotherapy, best surgery, and best radiation therapy from the best doctors in the world and the best hospitals in the world. Did my attitude and willpower have a role in healing me? Did my planning the care have a role in my healing and beating cancer? Did I get liberation from cancer? I do not know exactly the answer to these important questions and will never know. I want to believe that I did have a role in my recovery. Am I blessed and grateful to be alive and be 'cancer-free' today? Of course, yes! Did I get better because I was lucky? Definitely, yes! Did my doctors heal me? Most definitely, yes! Did my diet heal me? Yes! Did yoga heal me? Yes! Did my practice of faith heal me? Yes! Did God heal me? Certainly, yes! Did the light of the lights in me burn cancer? Yes! Did that 'One', 'Infinity', 'truth', 'fearless', 'enemy-less', 'power that is neither born nor dead', 'self-effulgent', 'eternally infinite truth' (cross-reference: Ik Onkar) that transcends everything we know and don't know, transcends everything we feel in any of our sensory organs, transcends mind or intellect heal me? Of course, yes! I want to believe that everything that I did and did not do, everything that happened to me and did not happen to me, whatever I received and did not receive must have played a role in healing me. In addition to chemotherapy, radiation, and surgery, every drop of water I drank, every bit of air I inhaled, every bit of food I ate (some may call it a cancer prevention diet, even though I cannot claim it), every positive thought that went through my mind, every minute of healing meditation I did, every prayer that I did and every prayer people did for me must have helped. All these are part of holistic cancer care. The space I was surrounded by, the friends and family I was surrounded by helped me heal. (Ayurveda, the ancient Indian medical philosophy, is based on the philosophy that the five elements, the air, water, earth, fire, and ether, determine and dictate our health and healing. That is what I am referring to. This principle is valid in modern medicine today as well.)

I had radiation and chemotherapy initially, followed by surgery and then more chemotherapy. I had to undergo another surgery after six months of having the initial surgery, not for cancer but to undo my ileostomy (where the terminal small intestine is directly connected to the outside through a hole in the right lower part of my tummy so the feces come out to a plastic bag that is attached to the skin) and re-establish the 'plumbing' of my intestines so I could have bowel movement through the normal passage.

Starting immediately thereafter, I had to deal with fecal incontinence. I changed my diet. I took medicines to slow down my bowel movements, tried medicines to solidify my stools, restricted fluid intake to solidify my stools, did Kegel maneuver to strengthen my anal sphincter, took biofeed-back to dictate, and coordinate my anal sphincter, meditated and prayed.

I went to temples and climbed mountains to visit certain Hindu temples and holy sites. I went to the famous St Mary's (St Michael's) church in Mahim, Mumbai, to pray. I also went to Haji Ali Dargah, a Muslim shrine in Mumbai. I prayed and took a dip at the holiest of the places for the Sikhs, the Golden Temple in Amritsar, India, and I also prayed at Saint Peter's Basilica in Vatican City. I have prayed at Bodh Gaya, where Buddha was enlightened, and I have worshipped at Isse, the holiest place for the Shintos of Japan. I prayed, chanted mantras and holy prayers, sang devotional songs (bhajans), and studied scriptures. My belief, based on studying scriptures, that I am a part of the infinite consciousness, just like a wave of an ocean, gave me immense strength to heal. That I am part of this infinite consciousness was very comforting, very healing, very soothing, very peaceful, very liberating, very enlightening, and very empowering. Knowing that I am the truth and part of the infinite truth was very empowering. The knowledge that I am a mini world (microcosm) that is inseparable from the infinite world (macrocosm) was very empowering. The knowledge that the single eternal, infinite truth that is fearless, loving, birthless, deathless, and timeless manifests in me was very peaceful and empowering.

My body suffered a lot of pain from colon spasms and ended up with intestinal obstruction about five years after having the initial surgery. When I was very close to having a major surgery by one of the best surgeons in Dallas, Dr. Alejandro Mejia of Methodist Transplant Institute, I changed my bowel management program by one hundred and eighty degrees in the opposite direction and have been doing it since then. That has served me well since then and has helped me work as a full-time physician with almost no pain and better bowel control. I am still on the same bowel program, and this program has tremendously improved my quality of life. I always believed that everyone has a unique story. That is why I wrote my story, which has been successful so far and worthy of sharing with you. I thank God for scripting my story with the hope that this will help at least one more human being, hopefully, more.

I am a sports fan. I have been part of sports teams as a hobby during my youth and sometimes have played the captain's role in our team. Sports have taught me to fail, fall, rise, and succeed. I have learned more from watching teams fail and succeed and also from listening to post-game interviews of both winning and losing captains along with coaches. I have analyzed why winning teams win and losing teams lose even though both teams are usually extremely good and are so close to winning. Usually, the difference between the winning and the losing team is very little. But that 'little' difference is very impactful.

Even though there is some finite element of luck or divine blessing, to a large extent winning is not an accident. It is usually an outcome of discipline, studying, planning a strategy, determination to win, positive psychology, confidence, proper guidance/coaching, practice, practice, and practice with equanimity of mind and unveiling the flow of divine infinite power within us at the right time and right place.

This is true for both team sports and individual sports. Even individual sport is a team sport involving multiple players in the background. Surviving cancer is very similar to team sports, which involve all these elements. Having said this, most of this does not come with a script, just like there is often no script for winning a game once you are in the field. You have to play the game as the situation demands. But if one incorporates the above-mentioned components like planning, determination, confidence, guidance, and practice in his/her life to strategize a win, the right decisions fall into place at the right time. Divine blessings help us take the right steps and make the body heal to culminate as a healed individual.

This book is a script of what I did to undo cancer and what happened to me. I have to admit that I did not have the whole script with me planned out when I was diagnosed with cancer. In fact, the diagnosis of cancer is very sudden and accidental in most situations. It does not come with a script for anyone. Talking to people, talking to doctors, reading books, and contemplating helps come up with a plan. That's what I did in my life too. The book is about how I took to the fight against cancer as the final game of my life. But I was not playing it alone. The entire team consisted of doctors, nurses, family, friends, relatives, supporting staff, and each and every one who helped me plan and play the game, which boosted my confidence to thrive through the journey.

I worked all day on that Wednesday in October 2004. I got many phone calls through the night and had to come early on Thursday morning to see four new patients I was called to see. In addition, I saw my usual load of patients in the hospital so I could have the colonoscopy at 1:00 p.m. I my wife and two of my close physician friends (Raju and Sumit) were told immediately after the colonoscopy that I had a mass (polyp) in the rectum. Looking back, it feels strange that my friends, Raju and Sumit came for my colonoscopy. My friends immediately had a strong suspicion that it was cancer. It took a few hours for me to sink in. I was probably not that sharp after recovering from sedation. Moreover, I never suspected that I could have cancer at that time. At the age of 41, I was not supposed to get cancer, or so I thought. Indeed, cancer of the colon or rectum is uncommon at that age. Cancer of the colon and rectum is uncommon among Indians. But I had lived outside India for 11 years by then. Cancer of the colon-rectum is more common among meat eaters, and I was not an avid meat eater, even though I had eaten some chicken and fish in my life. The next day at 11:00 a.m., I knew I had cancer! My life changed within 24 hours from being a busy, exuberant doctor to a new 41-year-old patient with cancer! There was some emotion, as you could expect in the family. My wife called her mother in India within a minute! What do people think when they find out someone has cancer? Death! It is common to think of death when one is diagnosed with cancer. At least, that is what most people think. But that was not what I was thinking. I hope, and I think, that is not what most patients are thinking when they have a new diagnosis of cancer. What will happen to my young kids if I die? My wife was a 35-year-old homemaker; what would happen to her if I died? These were some of the questions people were thinking about and some were asking. But I was thinking of living. I was thankful that I did not have kidney failure since I see that problem every day in my patients. Over the next few days, I realized that it was my obligation to my kids and family for me to survive cancer. I felt that I was responsible for taking care of them. Over the next few days, all I knew was that I wanted to beat cancer, and I knew that my best chance to win was to play the most comprehensive battle the very first time and to play it as though I was playing the 'world cup finals', as though, that was my last and the only game left.

I have empathy and admiration for those who are going through cancer treatment. But my advice to you is to challenge cancer in you, be humble, be strong, be competitive, be the spark to enlighten yourself, be the spark to ignite the fire in you to burn cancer in you, be positive and scientific, be the fire to provide light to your healthy immune cells and burn one cancer cell at a time at a pace faster than your cancer cells multiply and finally extinguish cancer in you. You will be left with only healthy cells, you will be left with only divine strength, you will be left with only the healthy 'YOU', you will be left with the 'Infinity' in you! You will realize that your body is not the real you and hence cancer does not belong to you. Your mind is also not the real you. The real 'you' is the infinite consciousness, which is infinitely powerful, immortal, and omnipotent.

'I recovered because I got the best chemotherapy, best surgery, and best radiation therapy from the best doctors in the world and the best hospitals in the world. I followed holistic comprehensive approach to my health and also seeked spiritual healing. And, I had THE POWER OF INFINITY! You have it too! It is for you to unveil it!'

Note: It would mean a lot to me and help many people undo cancer if you leave an honest review at amazon.com.

SECTION 2: SURVIVING CANCER

Chapter One
My Life Before Cancer

I was born in rural India in the southern part of the country along the west coast. The place is in the Udupi district, which is famous for Udupi Sri Krishna Temple and Udupi vegetarian food. It is close to Mangalore, a hub of educational institutions and hospitals. The place is known to have 100% literacy, greenery, beaches, allopathic and ayurvedic medical schools, treatment centers, temples, a melting pot of different faiths such as Hindus, Christians, Muslims, Jains, Buddhists, Sikhs, and others, and people from different parts of the world. I was born in a big family known in the area, but not many in the area including us knew that we were quite poor. We had few school teachers on the maternal side of the family; my three maternal uncles came up the hard way in life after moving to Mumbai and ended up becoming a lawyer with a Master's degree, an engineer with a doctorate, and a surgeon respectively. My parents were financially poor. My father was an agriculturist and my mother was a homemaker. For complicated and accidental reasons beyond the scope of this book, I grew up with my two brothers, two sisters, my mother, and my maternal grandparents. My father lived in his family home with his widowed sister and a few other family members. He visited us once or twice a month to our delight, usually two to three days at a time. Mother, I, and all my siblings lived with my father's side of the family along with my father during the summer and monsoon holidays for two to three months of the year. The reason for such a strange living arrangement was not due to any kind of fight, or problem with breaking the law or arrangement between my parents, it just happened for certain family needs!

My mother and my maternal grandmother were very hard working and influenced my life at an early age. My grandmother was a habitual and compulsive giver (donor). She would give when she had nothing to give. She would ask for things that she did not have so she could give them away. She would offer food to random people who would walk by our house. If someone died in the neighborhood, especially if a woman lost her husband, she would go and stay with them without an invitation for few weeks and cook for them and do their chores. In other words, she was a habitual and compulsive helper and an epitome of love and giving. My mother was a notch up in working hard. Even though there are certain norms as to what men do and what women do in the farms, there was hardly anything that she would not do if the need arose. The only task she never did was plow the land. I think I learned to love unconditionally from my grandmother and to work hard from my mother. Because of our strange family situation, I spent less time with my father. He was an extreme disciplinarian in the family and I was scared of talking to him till I joined medical school at the age of 17 years. We never had any conversation with him. His word prevailed. My father had zero tolerance for untruth and that is the inheritance I got from him. That is his biggest legacy.

My eldest brother, Kishore, left for Mumbai to work after passing the seventh grade. He simultaneously went to school to eventually graduate from college and also have a post-graduate diploma in industrial catering. He was a natural leader from school days. He was a giver like my grandmother; a hard worker like my mother. He played the role of a father in my life in many ways. He crafted my life. He was my guide, financer, cheerleader, and everything. I have another brother, Ashok, and two younger sisters, Asha and Shakku, all of them are very loving and I am very close to all of them. Ashok used to work harder than I did. I used to feel that I did not have as much stamina as he did. I spent more time with him than any of my other siblings. I watched him work harder than me, play better cricket than me, swim way better than me. His friends were my friends too. He was taller and stronger than me. He was very bold and learned to cycle without asking my parent's permission, something that I did not dare do. He taught me to work hard, he taught me to swim, he taught me to uphold the truth. He would work even if he was not well. His justification was that he may not be able to work the next day if he got sicker and hence would work as much as he could even if he was not at his best. He was uncompromising when it came to justifying and supporting truth and justice.

My sisters Asha and Shakku, both are very loving. Asha lives in India and gets the credit deservedly for taking care of my grandparents and my parents. She should get more credit for what she does. Sometimes I have to remind her that she did and does more for the family than the rest of us even though all her siblings may have more material wealth. My youngest sister, Shakku lives in the US and has walked with me through my journey of cancer. She has been the rock-solid pillar of support for me. Shakku was the darling of the house during her early childhood. She was extremely good at studies, went to medical school in India by sheer perseverance, and became a pediatric anesthesiologist in the US. She feels responsible for my healthcare and takes that very seriously, which has been very helpful to me and my wife. Since the time I had cancer, she has also helped many people with cancer in different ways that I could not imagine one could do. Sometimes I feel that it has become her passion in life. She has inherited a lot of good qualities from my maternal grandmother. During my school days, my third uncle graduated from medical school as a valedictorian and became a well-known doctor. I think I was very proud of being his nephew when I was in school. I think my doctor uncle, Dr. Sugandh Shetty influenced me to be a doctor even though I do not remember seeing him much when I was a child.

How were my school days? I had a normal childhood. I was good at mathematics and science. I used to play the game of cricket till I joined medical school. When I was in school, I did not think that I could afford to attend medical school. But my brother, Kishore told me not to worry about fees even though he was heaped under loans. My second uncle (Dr. Vasanth Shetty, Ph.D.) told my brother that he would support me if necessary. Even though I did not have to take help from him, getting assurance of support was very important for me and my brother. My third uncle, Dr. Sugandh, helped me financially and in many other ways till my brother became more comfortable with his finances. Later he helped me get an interview for residency in the US. I am very grateful to him for helping me at very crucial points in my life. Once I joined medical school, since I had to focus on studying and be good among the very good students from all over the world, I quit playing cricket. I had to transition to living among students from big cities and those from more affluent families. Even though I quit playing cricket, my interest in sports has continued and I watch various sports very closely and have learned a lot from them.

I don't remember having lofty dreams. I wanted to be the best that I could be. All I knew was that I did not have any inheritance to rely on and hence had to make a living on my own. The only way I knew of making a living was to study hard. I did not come from a family with a business background, even though we have become entrepreneurs of some degree over time. I just wanted to be a very good doctor and I wanted to be able to support my family. One of the challenges of growing up in the rural world without TV, radio, computers, personal vehicles, and phones was that I had not known my potential. For that reason, my dreams were very limited. I was like a frog within a well. I could only see my little world within the well. As I grew up, I saw the bigger world and grew with it. The more I grew, the more I saw and I grew further.

In India, one can go to medical school after twelfth grade. I was able to get admission to a very good school called Kasturba Medical College, Manipal in the southern part of the country. When I got admission to medical school at the age of 17 years, I was malnourished and had not attained the growth spurt of puberty and hence I was very little. Once when I was going to medical school by bus, the bus conductor thought I was in eighth grade! We had to struggle to pay for the fees. It was usual to mortgage my mother's jewelry to get a short-term bank loan to pay the fees on time. Later, my brother Kishore would pay off the loan and release my mother's jewelry. Mr. Ramachandra Shetty and Mr. Shantaram Shetty at the Vijaya Bank were very supportive of me and made things as smooth as possible for me. Mr. Shantaram Shetty, the bank manager, was very helpful in getting me a bank loan at a very low-interest rate based on low family income. He would also see me after bank hours in his house so I did not have to miss classes during office hours. My uncle, Dr. Sugandh Shetty also helped me financially till my brother, Kishore became a little more stable financially. I was also fortunate to secure Smt. Sitabai Godbole Scholarship from Syndicate Bank for three successive years and that was very helpful. Later my cousin, Mr. Sundar Shetty from Pune also helped me financially at a very critical time.

I had to get used to students from different parts of the world, who spoke really good English in different accents and were a lot more affluent. Even though I studied in the English medium in the eleventh and twelfth grades, I could not speak the language fluently. I only had one pair of pants and a shirt. I did not know that clothes had to be ironed. So, I used to wear wrinkled shirts and pants. My pants were very tight and sometimes the zipper used to come off in public to my humiliation. I did not have leather shoes. I had a pair of plastic sandals that were heavily used up. I later bought a pair of canvas shoes and rubber slippers. One of my lecturers used to make fun of me when I used to attend anatomy dissection hall in slippers. In twelfth grade, I was the salutatorian in my school and was the topper in science and mathematics subjects. But when I went to medical school, I realized that many had done better than me in the twelfth grade. We also had a few students from the US, South Africa, Malaysia, and other countries who were college graduates. Culturally, medical school was very different. I had to get used to young men and women sitting next to each other in the classroom, people having boyfriends and girlfriends, and eating breakfast while walking to the classroom. I had to quickly adjust to different languages, different slang, and accents of English. Despite all the adjustments, at that young age, there was no dearth of confidence in me. In fact, I am not sure if it was confidence. *I just did not compare myself with others and I did not let others judge me. This quality of mine has served me well in my life.* I lived in my own world trying to learn some English accents by twisting my tongue, which did not work! Since my father had a friend in the college town, Late Mr. Diwakar Shetty, he put me in a different dorm (hostel) to avoid ragging, also called bullying by the senior students, usually sophomores.

Mr. Diwakar Shetty was a very soft-spoken, humble, and gentle soul and I had and still have a lot of respect for him. He was my local guardian in many ways. I would never be able to pay back his favors. I really felt protected by him and never got bullied because I knew him. I used to refuse to even get verbally abused by the senior students who eventually became my friends. I did well in the first year of medical school. In my second year, much to everyone's surprise and my disappointment, I did not do as well as I was expected to do. This led to a lot of turmoil in my mind. To rebuild myself and my mindset, I subscribed to a magazine called, 'Competition Success Review' and it really helped me focus on my efforts and not the outcome. I also read a few verses of the sacred Hindu scripture, Bhagavad Gita, and picked the most famous verse from the second chapter. It taught me to focus on my efforts without taking ownership of the fruit of action. It helped me to be happy with my good actions and accept with grace whatever result that followed. The same verse stresses on not giving company to inaction and the same chapter later also stresses on being focused and having dexterity in action.

I think it was my friend Dr. Vittal Nayak, who eventually became an ophthalmologist, who told me about this great teaching. In 1983, I, along with everyone in the world, had the opportunity to witness the 'Infinity' of Indian cricket, Kapil Dev, who won the World Cup cricket championship for India. Kapil Dev was a true servant leader who believed in things that nobody in his team or the cricket fraternity believed. He convinced his team members that he had the team that could beat any team in the world, he led from the front, showed some extraordinary skills that nobody knew he had in the field, and eventually won the championship trophy for India. I learned a lot from him, the art of believing in myself, the art of servant leadership, believing in infinite potentials that we have, and infinite ways of manifesting that 'Infinity' in us. Thank you, Mr. Kapil Dev, for influencing thousands of us who have never met you in person, but you inspired us to unveil 'Infinity' and manifest it. I eventually did well in college and again graduated from medical school as the salutatorian! I missed being the valedictorian by a 0.057 percent difference in my score!

I studied further in other cities in India and Canada before I moved to the US to become a nephrologist, a specialist in kidney diseases. Dr. Amritlal and his brother and Late Dr. Sudhakar Shetty were very helpful later to help me obtain more educational loans. Mr. Damodar Shetty in Mumbai was another person who helped me make some critical career decisions in Mumbai. After completing my training in nephrology in Mumbai, I got married. In my in-laws' opinion, the yardstick for a successful doctor was to be like the famous cardiac surgeon, Dr. Devi Shetty. He is a very gifted surgeon with amazing surgical and entrepreneurial skills and is now the CEO of Narayana Health, a conglomeration of many hospitals in India and one in the Cayman Islands. He has mastered the skill of quality and affordable medical care for large masses of patients in India. He indeed was and still is the 'Infinity' in his field. I could never become like him. I never had the vision nor the skills he had. I had my own limited vision, which was different from his. After seeing famous doctors in Mumbai, I developed the desire to go abroad and learn peritoneal dialysis, a treatment that I did not have an opportunity to learn in India. I was fortunate to get that opportunity to work with Late Dr. Dimitrios George Oreopoulos in Toronto, Canada. He was one of the greatest experts in the field of peritoneal dialysis and one of the nicest human beings I have worked with. He was the 'Infinity' in his field. He has left a lot of impressions in my life. Dr. Oreopoulos fitted into the meaning of 'Guru' and not just a teacher. Guru is more like a mentor, a person who teaches you skills but also teaches life skills to become a successful person and a good human being. Besides peritoneal dialysis, I learned the skill of compassionate medicine, end-of-life care, unconditional love to your family and students, and serving the community at large from Dr. Oreopoulos.

I learned to write research papers and give credit to all the contributors to the papers from him. I was getting paid reasonably well in Canada as a trainee and I was under the impression that I would be able to save enough funds to feel comfortable to start a Nephrology practice in Mumbai. If I really wanted to, my brothers and in-laws would have helped me establish an office in one of the suburbs of Mumbai. But like I said earlier, as I grew my plans grew. I wanted to be in the best of the hospitals in Mumbai. But I did not think I had the funds to live closer to a big hospital in Mumbai. I also felt that the Canadian fellowship did not give me any acronyms like FRCP or Diplomate of the American Board of Internal Medicine in my business card unless I did internal medicine training in the US. I just felt that I did not have enough credentials at that time to get privileges in one of the major hospitals in Mumbai and be the best. Hence, I decided to go to the US to further my studies and get more degrees and acronyms on my business card. But I also never tried hard to establish myself in Mumbai. I know friends who went back to India with those credentials and have done extremely well. I just found the easier route. After completing my training in the US, I just found it easier to establish myself in the US and eventually chose to continue to live here with my wife and children. We spent the initial six and a half years in Detroit before we moved to Dallas, Texas to live closer to my sister.

During my life in the US, the sports lover in me fell in love with the game of basketball and started appreciating the Michael Jordan and Phil Jackson combination of the Chicago Bulls followed by the Shaquille O'Neal, Kobe Bryant, and Phil Jackson combination of the Los Angeles Lakers. Both teams were pursuing 'Infinity!' At the end of my third year in Texas, I was about to become a shareholder in our medical practice when I was diagnosed with cancer. Life has been different since then filled with a lot of pain and pleasure, ups and downs, gratitude, prayers, learning, and healing in pursuit of 'Infinity'.

Chapter Two

How It All Started

I was 41 years old leading a regular life with my family. One day, all of a sudden, I was told I had cancer. I had to undergo radiation, chemotherapy followed by extensive surgery in the abdomen and anal region. I was told about a high possibility of needing a colostomy (feces coming out to a plastic bag from the belly) after the surgery that may be permanent. The doctor said that being young might mean that cancer can be aggressive. That happened in October 2004! Life changed for me in a matter of a moment!

The summer of 2004 was a usual summer for us. We had gone to India to visit family. When I came back, I found myself having frequent bowel movements in the mornings. It is not that unusual to have diarrhea after traveling to a tropical country. I got treated for traveler's diarrhea. I was a little better, but I still had to go to the restroom twice most mornings. There would be a sense of incomplete evacuation of the rectum after the initial bowel movement requiring me to go again. Looking back, that is a classic symptom of something partially obstructing the rectum! But in medicine we have a saying, 'Common things happen commonly, uncommon things happen uncommonly'. And cancer of the rectum is not common at the age of 41 years. I had lost two pounds of weight during that summer and fall. I attributed that to my stress of both my sons developing pneumonia that September within a month. I remember my son asking me once, "Dad, how come you never fall sick?" My turn was just around the corner!

Sometimes, my stool had little dark streaks. It probably was blood in hindsight. The symptom was bothering me enough to see a gastroenterologist. He did a rectal examination that was painful. A rectal exam is uncomfortable; it is not supposed to be painful. Moreover, there was blood in the doctor's examining finger. He scheduled colonoscopy appropriately since he was suspecting some inflammatory bowel disease. I scheduled the procedure in about four to six weeks since I had to attend the American Society of Nephrology conference, which is a premier annual conference in my field. But both my friends, Raju and Sumit, somewhat insisted that I should not wait that long. Hence the colonoscopy was rescheduled earlier.

Two days before the diagnosis, I worked all day and night. I also worked the day before and had a colonoscopy at 1:00 p.m. The doctor who did the colonoscopy was shocked to see what he saw. Before he woke me up from anesthesia, he asked a colorectal surgeon to see it with his own eyes. After the procedure, he showed me a picture of a large polyp in the distal part of my colon, the rectum. He said that it can become cancerous. When I asked him the percent chance of it becoming cancer, he said '50%' and walked away. My thinking may have been fuzzy after recovering from sedation since it did not occur to me that the picture was looking like cancer. Nobody was suspecting cancer before the procedure and hence I was not even entertaining that diagnosis. Both my physician friends, Raju and Sumit knew it right away. Raju called my sister, Shakku in Houston and apparently, both cried on the phone. I also spoke to her that night and told her what the doctor said. I also told my colleagues that I was not going to come to work the next day.

Before the colonoscopy, I was dreading having a diagnosis like ulcerative colitis. But this was much worse. Normally we ask patients to come back for a follow-up in a week or two after such procedures to discuss the biopsy results. Being a nephrologist who does the biopsy of the kidneys, I knew that we can have the preliminary results of the biopsy in four to six hours. I do not remember if I was able to get proper sleep that night. I waited till 9.30 in the morning the next day and then called the pathologist for the report like I do as a physician. Little did I realize that I was a patient here in this instance! The pathologist was very gracious with me however and did not remind me that I am a patient. Pathologists don't give the reports to the patients directly since they don't get to meet patients. He told me that I should be able to get the report later in the morning. Normally pathologists interpret the biopsy slides under the microscope and give the result to the doctor who performed or requested the biopsy and whoever requested the biopsy delivers the result to the patient.

At around 11:00 a.m., my phone rang. It was my gastroenterologist who performed the colonoscopy and biopsied the tumor/polyp. That was the most dreaded phone call I have ever received in my life! He told me that I had cancer! There was no mincing of words. He was direct and to the point. This is not how 'bad news' is delivered to patients normally. But since I was a physician who already was expecting 'bad news' and since I was requesting the report right away, no time was wasted in giving me the news. If I were not a physician, I would have been asked to come to the office with a family member to discuss the results one or two weeks after the procedure. I got the results in the most efficient way. In a minute, I became a cancer patient. A 41 years old doctor in the prime of his career in the US suddenly became a cancer patient. Within a matter of seconds, from being a doctor who worked hard to prevent the sick from dying, I became a patient with cancer who had to find ways to survive. I had to look straight into the eyes of the God of Death to get out of my way. A few years later, my father-in-law told me that the God of Death came to me and then realized that he made a mistake, spit me out, and went away!

When I asked my doctor what the next step was, he said that I had to get an endoscopic ultrasound and a CT scan. I requested for the tests to be done at the earliest. So both the endoscopic ultrasound and the CT scan were done on the same day.

My wife and I remained briefly silent in shock! I hugged my wife and she cried! My extended family was all informed; my wife called my mother-in-law who also spoke to me. I informed my sister Shakku in the US. I could not reach my eldest brother Kishore on phone and then I informed my second brother, Ashok. I did not want to shock my elderly parents and since my other sister, Asha lived very close to my parents, I did not want to tell her as well, at least not so soon. But of course, news travel fast, and Shakku, could not keep it to herself and told Asha in a few days.

The endoscopic ultrasound showed that the tumor had not spread to the neighboring structures. That was relieving! I had the CT scan soon thereafter. I was not ready to wait for 24 hours to get the CT scan results since that was an extremely important test to determine the extent of the disease and hence my fate. In other words, a CT scan would tell me if the tumors had spread to the local lymph nodes, other surrounding structures, and the liver. If rectal cancer has already spread to the liver, you are done in most cases! The prognosis is poor except in rare situations if the cancer is spread to one small part of the liver, which can sometimes be surgically removed with good results.

I walked from the CT scanning table to the film reading room where the radiologists interpret the CT scan. The radiologist kindly reviewed my CT scan images with me and determined that the tumor had not spread. It was nerve-wracking to see my own images, but it was worth the moment since I got good news right away. When I hugged my friend Raju after getting the good news that the tumor was localized, the radiologist apparently gave a strange look to us according to Raju. She may have thought that we were a gay couple! But I couldn't care, of course. It was a relief to know that my cancer was localized. It was indeed a long day for me. Being a doctor in the same hospital probably helped me get the final diagnosis two weeks earlier than it would have taken elsewhere. These are some small perks for being a doctor, knowing the people, and knowing the system. After a few months, I remember my oncologist telling me that I was trying to beat the system. Yes, I was! Why not? I was just being efficient. I was not hurting anybody! It happens in every field. I heard that more than 80% of the jobs are not advertised. They are offered to known people if they are considered good. In the real estate world also, the best of the deals are gone before they are published.

In 2004, my cell phone was not as 'smart' as it is today. There were no iPhones or smart and fancy Android phones! There was no facetime! My phone ran out of battery and I knew that my family members may have been trying to reach me. It must have been hard for my wife to be by herself at home alone. She was suggested by her mother to go to my friend Raju's house and be with his wife Jyothi. As soon as the kids came home from school, she went to Raju and Jyothi's house where all my close friends gathered. There was some panic among my family members on my side and my in-laws in India. I don't know if anybody was trying to reach me. I was not reachable because my phone battery was dead and I was not home! The idea of being not reachable to my family members made me very uncomfortable. Raju drove me from the hospital to his house.

I was very tired and exhausted! I laid down for some time in Raju's bedroom and cried briefly while hugging my wife. All the friends were sitting in the family room. When I felt a little better after about 15 minutes,

I walked to the family room, stood behind the sofa so I could see everybody, and delivered my 'state of cancer' address! I told them what I knew about the extent of the disease. I told them that I wanted to lead a 'normal appearing' life. I requested my friends not to visit my house every day and not to bring food daily. I told them that it would help me feel closer to normal and recover faster if life went on normally. I thanked them and asked them to help our family when we asked for help. I assured them that I would ask for help if I needed it.

When Raju asked me to have dinner in his house, I refused and insisted that I should be home as soon as I could. I told him that I did not mind taking food from his house and eating at my house. I did exactly that! I just wanted to be at my house and be reachable and feel connected to my family living far from me, and deeply concerned. I almost felt that I was hiding from them. I felt that I was obliged to remain available for them to ask me questions and know more about what was wrong with me.

I invited my oncologist friend, Maryada Srinivas Reddy to my house that same night to talk to him about what to expect and also to explain to my sister in Houston about my situation. It was very relieving to talk to him. Srinivas has a very compassionate, but rational and honest way of discussing health issues, which was very helpful for me and my family.

I was busy planning my medical care and explaining to family and friends over the next few days. I soon realized that being a physician and the sole breadwinner of the family with a young wife and children, I had the responsibility to explain my disease to family members and also reassure them that I was going to get better. Instead of them consoling me, I had to console them. Since I am a physician, I had to do this! And for the extended family who could not see, touch, hug, and feel me, I had to do this over the phone!

Chapter Three

First Few Months With Cancer

Elements of planning the care, leadership, and team building

- **Acquire knowledge**

- **Mission: To come up with a multi-pronged attack on cancer as though I was playing the final game of the World Cup Finals**

- **Vision: Be cancer-free at five years and remain cancer-free after that**

- **Philosophy: You have one chance to come up with the best attack, and the first attack has to be the best one**

- **Strategy: A team approach to cancer survivorship; play like the final game of the World Cup series!**

The first thing you should do once you are diagnosed with cancer is to acknowledge that it has already happened to you. Once you accept the situation, you can think better about dealing with it and choose among the available treatment options. It is natural to ask questions like 'Why me?'. But that will not help you get better or go back in time.

There are a few important points one should keep in mind while dealing with cancer.

i. Team approach to cancer survivorship: Play like the final game of the World Cup series!

This chapter conveys the essential message of the book! Dealing with cancer or any serious problem takes a team approach. There are many parallels between dealing with cancer and playing a team sport. In this game of cancer survivorship, there are more players than just the patient and the doctor.

My brother Ashok had come from India to be with me during the surgery. While we were driving from Dallas to Houston to have the surgery at MD Anderson Cancer Center, he told me that dealing with cancer is like playing the game of cricket where the patient is the captain and multiple players are playing different roles. He was quoting a book written in Kannada. I don't remember the name of the book. But it made perfect sense to me, except that my game had begun three months before, and I had already made many decisions by then. I was already playing a team sport. I already had a great team, and he was an integral part of it.

Cricket is a team sport that is very popular in India and many other countries. The cricket team has 11 players and one substitute (backup) player. At a given time, two players from one team are batting, and 11 from the opposite team are fielding. The fielding team has a bowler who bowls the ball, a wicketkeeper, and nine fielders. Bowlers could be fast bowlers who bowl the ball as fast as 90-110 miles per hour, medium pacers, or spinners. Fast bowlers can throw a limited number of 'bouncers' that bounce at your body unpredictably, requiring you to respond within a fraction of a second to protect your body and your wicket. Even in the game of cancer survivorship, situations change suddenly, and you sometimes have to face challenging situations and make crucial quick decisions. I have had to make some tough and some easy decisions; some must have been good, and some not so bright. But all in all, the outcome was good.

My team and I must have made some vital right decisions and I have been incredibly blessed to do well in this game. In the game of cricket, depending upon how the ball comes to you, you have to hit the ball well to score if the ball comes easy to the bat, or gently hit the ball to defend if it is an in-swinger, or let the ball go if it is an out-swinger or 'duck' to protect your body from getting hit if the ball is a bouncer and comes on your body. Sometimes, you may try to hit every ball if there is a need to score fast in a minimal time.

The fielding team captain huddles with the team members periodically to strategize the game and encourage and empower team members. The captain gets to guide the bowler, pick the team, and decide which bowlers to employ, and they get to guide the fielding placement. Captains can take suggestions from the vice-captain and other players. And during break time, the captain also gets to talk to the coaching staff. On the batting side, the captain gets to decide the batting order. This batting order can suddenly be changed depending on the situation. Winning captains are known to take over the game during difficult situations. Do you remember Captain Cool, MS Dhoni, the captain of the Indian cricket team in 2011, suddenly changing the batting order and eventually helping India win the World Cup? Over 1.5 billion people are celebrating Team India winning the T20 World Cup 2024 as I update the book now. I remember the epic 'Infinity' moments of the series, starting from Rohit Sharma destroying the Australian bowling, Rishab Pant's flying catches, timely batting by Virat

Kohli and Axar Patel in the finals, magical spells of bowling by Jasprit Bumrah and Arshdeep Singh, crucial wickets by Hardik Pandya, and the epic catch by Suryakumar Yadav.

Indian cricket lovers know of Kapil Dev, Saurav Ganguly, Sachin Tendulkar, Yuvraj Singh, Rahul Dravid, MS Dhoni, Virat Kohli, Rohit Sharma, and Jasprit Bumrah, who could take over the game and devastate the opposite team under challenging situations. I have learned a lot from watching them on TV. I have also learned a lot while watching some legends in other sports. A few of those legendary players that I have followed and cherished watching are Michael Jordan, Shaquille O'Neal, Lebron James, Tim Duncan, and Kobe Bryant in basketball; Tom Brady, The Manning brothers, and Troy Aikman of American football; Roger Federer, Pete Sampras, Andre Agassi, Rafael Nadal, Novak Djokovic, Ramesh Krishnan, Rohan Bopanna, Sania Mirza, Martina Navratilova, Chris Evert Lloyd, Steffi Graff, Martina Hingis, Venus Williams, and Serena Williams in tennis; Diego Armando Maradona, Cristiano Ronaldo, and Lionel Messi in the soccer world. You all will have your list of favorites depending on your interests and age. There is also a team of head coaches, assistant coaches, managers, team doctors, physical trainers, and a selection committee. During the game of cricket, the captain is practically the coach, unlike other team sports like basketball and American football, where the coach is very involved on an ongoing basis.

In going through cancer treatment, I know I played the role of a captain. I may have played the head coach position as well, even though I had many coaches guiding me.

As a captain of the cancer survivor team, you have to build a strong team and manage your team. The team comprises the spouse, children, parents, in-laws, siblings, and other significant family members, friends, oncologists, radiation oncologists, surgeons, radiologists, anesthesiologists, pathologists, nurses, dieticians, spiritual guides, and others. Every member on this list has a unique role, and hence, the list is not in any order of importance.

In this list, you get to pick oncologist(s), radiation oncologist(s), surgeon(s), anesthesiologists, and sometimes radiologists and pathologists. You get to pick the friends who can help you. However, you don't get to decide who your family members are, although you get to decide whom to take help from depending upon the need and the available skills. Since I am an immigrant in the US, I had more friends living close to me than family members. I did not hesitate to take help from them.

I had friends who provided motivation, medical guidance, spiritual guidance, medical literature, strategic advice, help with taking care of children, and many who were supportive of me unconditionally with an abundance of love. Some provided transportation, and some helped with communication. I realized that more friends wanted to help me than I needed. But having so many people willing and wanting to help is a good situation. Most people in this world are good. I found out later that hundreds of people who knew me directly or indirectly prayed for me and wanted to help me. Some of them were friends or friends of friends, many were nurses and medical staff, and a lot of them were patients and their family members. They say, 'It takes a village to raise a kid'. In my case, it took a few villages to make me better. I don't know what worked, but here I am, working full time and writing this book many years after finding out that I had cancer and putting lots of leadership lessons into practice.

ii. Being the captain of the team

When you have cancer, you have to initially define your goals, opportunities, plan of care, backup plan of care, managing survival versus managing quality of life, and decisions about the quantity of life versus quality of life, managing the family and friends to maintain peace and harmony in your life and among your family members.

When you read the literature, focus on the survival rate, not the mortality rate. Know that there are survivors even in late-stage cancer. Know that you don't survive a certain percent when the literature says five-year survival is X, Y, or Z %. You either survive 100% or you don't. All you have to do is to 'survive 100%'. If 90% survive, you have to be in the 90% that survive. If 10% survive, you must be one of the 10%. You will still survive 100% and not 10%. You have to do everything to be on the surviving side. Those who survive do so either because they are lucky to have cancer that is very responsive to treatment or because they got the best care, or both. Often, there is an element of both. Those who don't do well do so either because they have cancer that does not respond well or because they did not get appropriate care, or because luck was not on their side. Often, there is an element of all the factors. Sometimes, patients respond to treatment but suffer from the consequences of treatment.

"Asking for help does not make you a loser. Surrendering to God does not make you weak."

As the captain of my team, I took on many responsibilities to help me win. I had to pick the best team that I could pick to give myself the best chance to win. First of all, I had to pick the medical team. When a patient is a non-medical person, the patient would be referred to either an oncologist or a surgeon. Since I was working in the same hospital where my cancer was diagnosed, I decided to choose my team of doctors after consulting a few good friends. I had a close friend who is an oncologist. After serious thoughts, research, and discussion with friends, I decided that my oncologist friend should remain my friend and a critical medical advisor.

I discussed with a senior colleague of mine to recommend the best oncologist in town. He suggested two in the same hospital I was working at and another at the nearby University of Texas Southwestern Medical Center. Even though all of them were highly qualified, I chose Dr. John Cox because I felt that I could participate better in my care plan decisions besides the fact that he was a very well-respected, knowledgeable, and humane physician.

"It is important to choose a physician with whom you can freely communicate and one who empowers you."

I was not ready to give up that opportunity to participate in my care because I had too much at stake. This approach worked for me, and others may take different approaches that could work as well.

"Don't go by the ratings of the rating agencies to pick your doctor."

It can be a daunting task to choose a doctor. I benefited from being a physician and knowing how the medical system works. I think I have insight into what works and what does not. In this era of easy informational exchange, some decisions are tough to make. Knowing at least one physician whom you trust to be your advocate can benefit you a lot. This physician does not have to be your friend. They can be your primary care doctor or a doctor from a specialty. One thing I would recommend against is that please don't go by the 'best doctor' list. While some excellent doctors get into this list, many campaign to be on such lists, and many win popularity contests for non-medical reasons.

Another thing to avoid is the reports from grading agencies. Grading agencies often have reports only from the disgruntled patients and none from the satisfied patients. I know some excellent doctors who have one (one of five) star ratings from one or two narcotic-seeking patients for refusing to prescribe such medications and no report from any other satisfied patients. When you google such doctors, all you see is those one-star ratings suggesting they are terrible doctors. Waiting time carries a lot of weight in patient satisfaction scores, and often, the centers of excellence have long waiting times. In my case, I was allowed to see my doctor at MD Anderson Cancer Center within two weeks of my diagnosis. I was an 'add-on' patient and ended up waiting around three hours to see my doctor the first time. I never complained, and I got the best care from this doctor who saved my life. As a physician, I focus on one patient at a time without thinking of my next patient and end up being late for patients later in the day. Even though I risk bragging, I guess I take excellent care of my patients. So the bottom line is, don't go by the ratings of the agencies to pick your doctor. Take help from your trusted doctor to pick other doctors.

iii. Building the INFINITY team that cannot fail!

Leadership and positive psychology are also important while dealing with severe obstacles in life. Cancer is simply the uncontrolled growth of abnormal cells. When the body functions normally, it regulates cell growth, manufactures new cells to replace the dead and dying ones, and then sends a clear signal to stop when enough cells have been produced. In the case of cancerous cells, the stoplight malfunctions, and the green light is always on, which means having masses of cells piling up and blocking normal regulation and functioning of the body.

As the cancer cells multiply, they form masses of cells known as tumors, which press against surrounding cells, causing damage and destruction to healthy tissues. Some tumors are distinct and well-defined; they are polite and keep themselves in their areas. Cancerous tumors, on the other hand, are rude and rebellious, directly invading their neighbor's space and breaking off from the mother tumor to travel through the bloodstream or lymph system to distant organs, where they create havoc. If the entire process is not controlled with various available treatments on time, it can lead to death.

One of the first things I did once I found out about my cancer was to know more about the disease in terms of treatment options and prognosis with the help of my medical friends and the available literature. As a medical person, I felt the need to do this. But this step is not that important because you want your doctor to make some of these decisions even if you are a doctor. Non-physicians should not try to make medical decisions and evaluate the medical literature on their own, even though they should acquire knowledge and ask relevant questions. I have seen some patients do poorly because they took it upon themselves to make all choices and not allow the medical team members to make the decision.

Be careful when you use Doctor 'Google'! Why would a software engineer make medical decisions? Would you like your doctor to fix your computer? Would you like your carpenter to repair your air conditioner? Put doctors to work. Let them do what they are trained to do. After studying for over 13 years after high school, they should know what they are doing. That does not mean every doctor is excellent. Just like any field, the skill set of the doctors varies, and you have to do some due diligence to choose the right doctor for you. It is hard even for doctors to choose their doctors. Just because something is published does not mean it is the right thing to do. Just because it is on the internet does not mean it is the proper treatment for you.

Having said this, it is hard to find out who is good and who is not. It is reasonable to request that your primary doctor help you choose the best doctor. But if you go to a tertiary care hospital in another city, it is hard to find out about the doctors. Sometimes, you simply have to assume that the best hospital will give you the best doctor. Even after knowing the medical literature, the treatment has to be individualized to you. Medicine is still an art that requires precision, knowledge, compassion, and common sense to get the best medical care, even though there is a lot of talk about artificial intelligence and big data helping make decisions and reducing medical errors. These technologies will indeed supplement and guide human intelligence. They may reduce medical errors, but I think there will always be a place for human intelligence to deliver the best personalized medical care.

iv. You have one chance to come up with the best effort and survive: The first chance is the best

Leadership and positive psychology again! When I was preparing and planning my treatment, I had no experience doing it since this was the first time for my family. But I knew a few things. The first point I knew was that the cure rate was not 100%. In fact, medical journals don't publish cure rates. They often publish cancer-free rates at five years. According to my reading, my chances of being cancer-free in five years were 80-90%. But my surgeon said that young patients could have more aggressive cancers, and hence my chances may be 60%. At the age of 41, this was not acceptable to me. Forget about 60%. Even a 90% chance of being cancer-free at the age of 46 years was not acceptable to me! I wanted it to be 100%. Later, the same surgeon told me before my surgery that these percentages do not matter much in a given patient. One patient does not get 60% or 90% cancer-free. A person becomes 100% cancer-free or 100% 'cancered' (I made up this verb!). He also told me that I had a good chance of doing well. The second point that I knew was patients don't do well if cancer comes back. It is harder to go back and resect it because of the scars from the first surgery. Surgeons don't like to do it if they can help it. Chemotherapy options for recurrent cancers are more aggressive, with more side effects and less success rate. The third point I knew was that different doctors treat patients differently since every patient with the same diagnosis is different in certain ways. Depending upon their overall health, their ability to tolerate the disease and tolerate treatment is different. Many times, centers of excellence are two or three years ahead of others. It matters more if it is the time of transition for a new treatment regimen to be the standard of care. Later, I realized that we were in such a phase in the evolution of the treatment of colorectal cancer. The other point is that I knew I was different in many ways. At the age of 41yrs, I was younger than most patients with rectal cancer. Rectal cancer is rare among Indians. Also, rectal cancer is more prevalent among meat eaters, and I was not one of them.

With all this information and mainly because I wanted to be 100% cancer-free forever, I wanted to put my best effort to give myself one best chance to be cancer-free. I was fortunate to be living not too far from MD Anderson Cancer Center, Houston, which is one the best places in the world to treat cancer. I was also fortunate to have my sister living in Houston. Her being a physician was helpful. Her friends were my friends, too. Hence, I felt I had a whole and parallel support system in Houston. That made the logistics a little easier. Fortunately, I found a divine soul in my Oncologist, Dr. Ajani, at MD Anderson. Dr. Ajani had two points to make. One, even though the oxaliplatin-based regimen was only approved for more advanced colorectal cancers at that time, he predicted that it would become the standard of care in a few years. The second point he made was that I should try my best to avoid permanent colostomy since it really affects the quality of life. He referred me to a surgeon, Dr. John Skibber, who was known for 'sphincter preserving' surgery to avoid a colostomy. Looking back, he indeed lived up to the expectations. Today I don't have a colostomy and I like it that way.

Dr. Ajani chose the chemotherapy protocol, and I was fortunate to find an oncologist in Dallas in Dr. John Cox, who was experienced in using these drugs and was comfortable administering an oxaliplatin-based regimen according to the recommendations from Dr. Ajani. So far, I had the best chemotherapy option chosen by the best oncologist I could find in the best cancer center in the world. I picked an excellent surgeon from the best cancer center in the world to give me the best chance to avoid a colostomy. My surgeon is traditional. Other surgeons try to improve anal continence by other surgical options such as the creation of a 'rectal loop' and/or doing minimally invasive surgery using robots and laparoscopes. At that time, I did not feel compelled enough to pursue these options since that would have complicated decision-making furthermore. Minimally invasive surgery has evolved in the last ten years, and I recommend exploring these options without compromising the quality of the surgeon. I feel I got excellent care from an outstanding surgeon.

Radiation therapy (Radiotherapy): I used to think radiation is just zapping the cancer tissue with X-rays. I had not done much research on it. But now I know that there are different kinds of radiation machines. The newer ones give radiation that is more targeted to cancer and minimize the damage to the surrounding tissues. So, it is up to you to do this research and ask your medical oncologist the right questions. But the easiest thing to do is go to the best center that you can go to. I don't know if the outcome would have been different, but I did not necessarily get radiation from the best machine available at the time. Most likely, it did not matter in my case. I do not know if I would have had better control of my anal sphincter if I had radiation from a more sophisticated machine because one of the side effects of radiation is collateral damage to the surrounding structures. The risk of radiation to the pelvis is damage to the anal sphincter and the nerves supplying it, making incontinence worse. There can potentially be some damage to the bone marrow that produces white blood cells, which can reduce the white blood cell count. Generally, this is of no consequence since there is bone marrow elsewhere. Radiation to the rectum can cause frequent rectal bleeding that can be a nuisance. Radiation damage to the rectum (called 'radiation proctitis' in the medical world) never causes severe bleeding, it just appears scary seeing your own blood! Theoretically, targeted radiation in the newer machines has the risk of leaving behind some cancer cells too.

v. Can a friend be your doctor? Yes, but!

Being a doctor comes with the luxury of knowing many other doctors. One of my closest friends happens to be a cancer specialist (oncologist). I called him home the day I was diagnosed. I had him talk to my wife and my sister. It was very important for me to have someone like Dr. Maryada Srinivas Reddy on my side. He is very calm, soothing, and, at the same time, objective. I was thinking of having him as my treating oncologist. I thought very hard. I talked to other friends and my wife. My wife wanted him to treat me. But one point bothered me.

At that time, I did not know how well or poorly I was going to do during my treatment. My thought was that I did not want to give him the burden of giving my wife the bad news if I were not to do well. There was also a fear that close friends could get emotional and lose the ability to be objective in difficult situations. The Texas State Board of Medical Examiners, the board that gives medical licenses, recommends not treating family members for the same reason. Even though I was not biologically related to Dr. Reddy, I was a close friend. Moreover, I felt that I would always have him on my side to help me make decisions related to my care if I chose another oncologist.

While I was thinking, I also asked him to think about whether he would be willing to treat me. He did independent research, consulted experts in the field in other parts of the world, and agreed to treat me. But I told him to remain as my friend and advisor. I may have momentarily disappointed him, but I felt right about my decision. I explained to him how and why I had made the decision, and he understood it well. There is no right or wrong answer here. I know of surgeons who have done open-heart surgery on their parents with successful results. Nobody complains when everything goes well, but if the outcome is poor, there will be many questions with difficult answers. I did not want my best friend to go through those risks. And I also did not want to lose a good friend if I did not do well. Remember my approach— I had one good chance to do well on the first attempt! As I said, I wanted to play like I was playing in the 'World Cup Finals.' And that is what I did. I chose him as my oncologist 'consultant,' and we did really well together. He has since stood as a strong pillar of support for me.

vi. How did I pick my doctors?

I decided to have two parallel systems. I knew that I had the luxury of having the best cancer hospital in the world, not too far from me in Houston. I was also fortunate to have my physician sister in Houston. That came with some ease of finding doctors in Houston and having a place to live. There is a bedroom in her house, the guest bedroom, referred to as 'Anup Mama's room' (*mama* means uncle) by my nephews!

What do I mean by having parallel systems? I had to have doctors in Dallas to go to. I knew that if I got sick suddenly, I would not be able to run to Houston. So, I had an entire team of doctors from various specialties in Dallas and another entire team in Houston. My good friend and colleague, Dr. Karl Brinker, helped me shortlist three oncologists in Dallas. I chose Dr. Cox out of them based on his excellent reputation within the Methodist Health System, Dallas, and not based on online surveys! I also weighed the ease of communication and negotiation of my choices with him compared to other doctors. Even though the other two doctors were also excellent, I did not have that comfort level to have free two-way communication with them. Freedom of choice and having a doctor who would listen to me was necessary, and Dr. Cox gave me that. After I started seeing him, I learned that he had some experience using oxaliplatin in advanced colorectal cancers, and he was willing to use it on me, as was suggested by Dr. Ajani from MD Anderson Cancer Center Houston. It was not experimental, but it was off-label use for the early stages of colorectal cancer, and some oncologists were not comfortable prescribing me this medicine since that was not FDA-approved for my stage. This made my life easier since I did not have to get chemotherapy in Houston. All I had to do was see my doctors in Houston and get a letter suggesting a treatment regimen. Dr. Cox would make some changes if he felt necessary, and I was able to get the infusions in his cancer center. Thankfully, I rarely had to negotiate treatment choices with him, but we had a great relationship, and we still do.

vii. Doctor, what are my chances?

It is a good practice to go through the statistics of survival rates and death rates. Initially, when I was reading the literature, I was focusing on percent survival. Generally, in oncology literature, survival is stated as two years of cancer-free survival and five years of cancer-free survival. It can be nerve-wracking when you are young. Here I was, 41 years old, and checking my two-year and five-year survival rates. I read literature suggesting that the odds of my five years surviving can be 70–90%. I was thinking that even a 90% survival rate is a 10% death rate in five years, and that was not good enough at the age of 41 years. Since I was young, my survival rate must be at least 90% if not 100%. Then, I asked my surgeon what my chances of survival were. He said that my five-year survival chance could be 60%. I told him that I read about it being 90%. I told him I was young and that I should do better! I almost felt entitled to do well. I caught myself negotiating for a better outcome! I caught the patient in me wanting to have better than the published outcome! I caught myself not wanting to be an average patient! I caught myself wanting to beat the odds!

He agreed that I am younger than most of the patients with rectal cancer but also said that, generally, cancer can be more aggressive in younger patients. I rested my case since I could not negotiate for a better-expected outcome! I knew I could come up with the best effort and action. But I could not control the outcome. Nobody can! But better news was coming.

Although it was a depressing visit for a few moments, I was too busy to be depressed. I had an appointment to have a 'port' placed in my chest the same day in Dallas. It goes into a big vein in the neck and gets tunneled under the skin to connect to a port in the chest wall. I realized there was no way I could fly back in time to get the port that day (it was a Friday). I was worried that delaying the port would mean delaying the chemotherapy that was going to be started the following Monday. But my oncologist told me that I could get the port and start chemotherapy the same day. Some advantages of being young, and knowing the people and the hallways in the hospital! We usually keep the days less busy for new patients by not having too many procedures/visits on the same day to reduce the physical and mental stress. But I did not mind it. My age and adrenaline surge helped me walk the long hallways of the hospital. I got the port placed the following Monday and started chemotherapy the same day.

Fast forward to a pre-operative visit with my surgeon before having the surgery. For localized rectal cancer, the routine standard is to get chemotherapy and radiation initially and wait for about six weeks for the area to heal (swelling to resolve) a bit before getting cut. My brother, Ashok, wanted to come with me to the pre-op visit, and I also wanted him with me.

Since my brother can be emotional, I was suggesting to him indirectly that I wanted to go for the surgery in a positive state of mind and that I did not want anybody to cry or say anything negative before the surgery. So I started preparing him by saying that the surgeon is excellent but very honest in telling things the way they are. I told him that sometimes the truth can be painful, but we don't have to worry and that I would do well. I went ahead and saw the surgeon after having a blood draw, anesthesiology visit, and MRI scan. The MRI scan would show the extent of the shrinking of my cancer after chemotherapy and radiation. I may have been a little nervous! I don't remember. Hey Rama! Hey Krishna! Hey, Mother Kali! Hey, Goodness Gracious! This time, my surgeon was so encouraging after he saw the MRI scan that showed significant shrinkage of cancer. He told me that all the cancer cells may have died.

The curious 'me' asked the same question again! I did not like his answer three months ago from the same doctor! Why would I ask that question again? Here I go again. Doctor, what are my chances? My doctor gave me such a good answer that I have been quoting him whenever my patients ask me similar questions. This is what he told me. "*Look, Anup! I can quote you a percentage.* **But that percentage is not going to help you. The only thing that will help you is if you do well.** *You are not going to survive by a certain percentage. Ninety percent survival chances look good, but it does not help if you are in the 10% that does not do well. A given patient will either* *survive 100% or not survive 100%."* And then he said the most important thing that I wanted to hear. He said, "I think you are going to do well."

I can't tell you how 'energizing,' 'enlightening,' and relieving this comment was for my family and me. This comment works in every field of medicine. When my patients ask what their chances of requiring dialysis are, I say a similar thing. I tell them that you are either going to be on dialysis 100% or you are not going to be requiring it at all. There is nothing in between. I do tell them that I will do everything that can scientifically be done anywhere in the world to avoid dialysis. Having said that, if I know a more certain answer, which we do often, I do tell them. I tell them either that 'there is a reasonable chance that you will not need dialysis in your lifetime unless something serious happens to you suddenly' or 'there is a high chance that you will need dialysis in your lifetime.'

viii. How vague or precise should doctors be?

I told you about my interaction with my main surgeon. It was a very pleasant one. He gave me facts, literature, and his expert opinion. That is what I expect from the doctors. I want them to know not only the current literature but also how that information applies to me in his hands in the setup that I am in. I was warned by a very good colon and rectal surgeon to make sure that I chose the best surgeon and not assume that I would get one just because of the hospital's reputation. You can have the best doctor in the best hospital (with the best of nurses, technicians, machines, radiologists, anesthesiologists, pain specialists, hospital administrators, and others), the best doctor in a mediocre hospital, or a mediocre doctor in an excellent hospital.

I indeed had the best surgeon in the world operating on me in the best hospital in the world. Sometimes, I see the 'googled' patients. With rare exceptions, I can help these patients interpret the information. The essential thing one should know is that you can put anything online. Not everything applies to a given patient even among the information published in medical journals. There are different journals and different kinds of publications. There are original articles, case reports (on one patient), case series (few patients), review articles, and editorials. Editorials and sometimes review articles carry the opinions of the authors. All kinds of publications carry cross-references to other articles, and the information can be misquoted or misinterpreted easily. My suggestion to patients who do a lot of independent research is to get help from their doctors to interpret the information. If you don't like what you hear from one doctor, take a second opinion. But please try not to be an expert in a field you are not. It can be dangerous to your health.

Just like it takes many years to learn a skill, it has taken many years of studying and experience for your doctor to be where they are. Just imagine how long it took for you to play a line on the piano or, sing a classical song or perform a classical dance. If you don't trust your doctor, go to a different one. Don't waste their time and yours. I went a little bit off track!

Another important point is to be ready to consent to a wider range of procedures just in case they become necessary. I signed consent to remove pretty much every organ in my pelvis! Thankfully, I only needed stents, which were removed after a few days of having surgery. (Please note that stents in the blood vessels of the heart and elsewhere cannot be removed once they are placed! But stents in the ureter can be. Sometimes they just come out on their own).

Once you are under anesthesia, they can't wake you up in the middle of the surgery to do more extensive surgery! So, it is better to consent to procedures that may become necessary at the surgeon's discretion once they open you up.

ix. Chemotherapy and radiation

Treatment of cancer involves surgery, chemotherapy, and radiation. I had all three modalities. The modality of treatment one gets depends upon the type of cancer. Some need only one of these modalities, and some need all three. For example, localized early colon cancer needs only surgery. In my case, I needed all three modalities. If one has extensive cancer, the goal of treatment may be palliative, and only chemotherapy or radiation may be recommended. If it is very extensive and life expectancy is very limited either because of cancer or because of other medical problems, only symptomatic management may be more appropriate. You have to decide whether treatment is better than cancer. If the tumor is very slow-growing and if it is felt that the cancer may outlive the person, not treating it may be a better option. It used to be a widespread practice not to treat chronic lymphocytic leukemia after a certain age. However, with newer treatment options and fewer side effects, most cancers are treated these days. In other words, it is better to discuss the care with the treating doctors and your family to determine the goals of care and then decide what approach is right for you.

Chemotherapy consists of administering medicines to kill cancer cells. These medicines are commonly administered into a vein. If the medicine irritates the vein, the patient will need a port placed in the chest that goes into one of the large veins in the neck. Some chemotherapy medicines can also be administered by mouth.

There are different kinds of radiation machines. The newer ones give radiation that is more targeted to cancer and minimizes damage to the surrounding tissues.

It is not unusual to face contradictory choices in cancer care. That puts you and your doctor between a 'rock and a hard place.' You become like the 'tongue caught between the teeth.' You simply have to trust your doctor in such situations. One example is that many chemotherapy medicines reduce the white cell count in the blood, which predisposes to infections. If the white count is very low, these patients need to take medicine to increase the white cell production. But one of the side effects of these drugs is that they can by themselves increase the cancer risk. In other words, a patient with cancer will be prescribed a drug that can increase the risk of cancer! That is an oxymoron! Isn't it? Here is another example. When the chemotherapy makes the white cell count go down, we have to stop the chemotherapy and hold it till the white cell count comes up. Similarly, if there is an active infection, we have to stop the chemotherapy till the infection gets better. This is not so much a situation of choosing from contradictory choices. Nevertheless, a patient with cancer does not like the interruption in the treatment. But doctors have to make those choices for the overall good of the patient. One of the common side effects of 5 fluorouracil that I got was frequent bowel movements. But the radiation to the rectal and anal region makes the area raw and painful. Thankfully, the rectum has no regular sensation except the stretch sensation. Since part of the area close to the anus has a sensation, having a bowel movement with a raw and inflamed rectum and anus is very painful. Imagine passing 'ropes' of stool over raw skin, another experience of raw denuded tongue caught between the sharp teeth! I had one of those painful nights with several painful bowel movements all night with blood in the stools. When I called my oncologist in the morning, he immediately reduced the dose of the chemotherapy medicine from seven days a week infusion to five days a week infusion. I was transiently sad and upset that the dose was reduced. I wanted my best chance to beat cancer and did not like the dose of medicine reduced.

Momentarily, I felt that I should not have called him! But I also knew that the pain during bowel movement was torture, and I knew that my doctor decided to help me. He played that balancing act of weighing the risk versus benefit and reducing the dose of anticancer medicine in the face of cancer to reduce a brutally painful side effect. Thank you, Dr. Cox, for lowering the dose of my medicine when I was literally crying during every bowel movement. That was a humane act of compassion from my doctor. That was a balancing act at its best by my doctor. I can still feel the pain that I had during every bowel movement with an inflamed, raw rectum and anus from radiation!

There are many medical situations where the correct choice is still being determined. There may need to be more data to help make decisions. In such situations, doctors may have to make decisions based on the science behind those treatment choices, their experience, and compassion. During the early part of my medical training, I was taught to commit to a diagnosis and treatment plan even in uncertain situations and make treatment decisions based on that. Some doctors ask the patients to make choices in such situations. Then there are some who provide all the information to the patients and also recommend one approach based on their scientific knowledge and experience they have after confessing what is unknown. I like the latter category of doctors, and I belong to that category.

x. Immunotherapy to treat cancer:

This part is taken from the website www.cancer.gov, and you can find more information there if you want to learn more.

"Immunotherapy is a type of cancer treatment that helps you fight cancer. The immune system helps your body fight infections and other diseases. It is made up of white blood cells.

How does immunotherapy work against cancer? As part of its normal function, the immune system detects and destroys abnormal cells and most likely prevents or curbs the growth of many cancers. Even though the immune system can prevent or slow cancer growth, cancer cells have ways to avoid destruction by the immune system. For example, cancer cells may:

-Have genetic changes that make them less visible to the immune system.

-Have proteins on their surface that turn off immune cells.

-Change the normal cells around the tumor so they interfere with how the immune system responds to the cancer cells.

Immunotherapy helps the immune system to better act against cancer. Immunotherapy can be administered by oral, intravenous, topical, and intravesical (into the urinary bladder) route"

xi. Side Effects of treatment

In his book, Lance Armstrong once said, 'In cancer care, side effects are guaranteed, but results are not.' There is a lot of truth to this statement. Chemotherapy medicines are usually very toxic medicines. Often, they not only kill cancer cells, but they also kill normal cells. That is why many of them lose hair, some develop painful ulcers in the mouth, some drop their white blood cell count, some get numbness in the feet, some develop infections, and others get some other side effects. Since we need white cells to fight infections, it makes them prone to serious infections.

It is essential to minimize visitors during chemotherapy to reduce exposure to infections. When you are on chemotherapy, your doctors may ask you to avoid uncooked fruits and vegetables. You may have to take some vaccines before starting some treatment. Your doctors may have to rule out and sometimes treat tuberculosis (TB) before starting certain medicines. Sometimes, you have to take some shots to increase the white blood cell count. The product label of some of these medicines will read that it may increase the risk of cancer, blood clots, or death. Why would your doctor prescribe something that would increase the risk of cancer or death when you already have one? That is because that risk is lower than the potential risk of not administering it.

Over the years, chemotherapy has transformed and has become more user-friendly, and side effects have come down. There are better medicines to control nausea, a common side effect. The medicines to combat nausea have become generic and affordable. There is also a new generation of drugs that are more focused on the target, hence having fewer effects on healthy cells. These have fewer side effects. Many of these are oral medicines. These medicines have a new line of side effects as well, which are not like the traditional side effects of chemotherapy medicines mentioned earlier, and hence, even the doctors may not be entirely familiar with these. To address the kidney-related side effects from chemotherapy drugs, a new sub-specialty called 'onco-nephrology' has evolved.

Many people getting chemotherapy wear masks. Masks are overrated. Masks protect you from the droplets of secretions that other people may cough on you. Masks protect others from getting an infection from your droplets of secretions when you cough. Masks do not prevent you from inhaling bacteria or viruses. Regular masks do not filter the air from these germs. Some special masks like N95 masks, if worn snugly without allowing the air to leak from the sides of the mask, will filter the air from bacteria to some extent. These masks are generally not worn by the patients since they are very uncomfortable to wear all day. They are usually worn by health care providers when they attend to someone with infections like tuberculosis or COVID-19 in the hospital. Hence, there is not much merit in wearing a mask at home. If anybody in the family is suffering from a respiratory tract infection, that person should wear a mask. It is reasonable for a patient on chemotherapy to wear a mask if someone in the family is coughing. The COVID-19 pandemic has taught us to reuse masks. Use your common sense to avoid wearing dirty masks. If anybody has a respiratory tract infection, it is better if that person stays away from the person on chemotherapy. The risk of acquiring infection is higher if the white blood cell count goes down after chemotherapy. White cell count does not go down after all the chemotherapy. Your oncologist will be able to tell you if your white cell count will go down. Standard chemotherapy for colon cancer generally does not reduce white count much, but those for breast cancer, lymphomas, and leukemias generally do. It depends upon the drugs that they receive. It makes sense to wear a mask if one cannot skip crowded environments such as the trains in Mumbai or the subways in New York City.

The COVID-19 pandemic has made us familiar with masks. There are different types of masks. To make it simple, three kinds of masks are frequently used. Regular cloth masks protect from inhaling droplets. These droplets come when a person coughs or laughs or breathes forcibly close to you. Surgical masks are made of cloth or paper in three layers. These masks also protect us from inhaling droplets more efficiently than regular one-layered cloth masks. Better masks are N95 or K95 masks. If worn properly and fitted right, these masks filter dust particles and bacteria. These are more uncomfortable to wear for prolonged periods. If you want to protect yourself in a dusty environment, you should wear an N95 or K95 mask. But if you are going to wear a mask for a prolonged period and if your white cell count is low, it is more practical to wear a surgical mask. It is a reasonable compromise knowing that these masks do not filter dust particles and bacteria.

xii. Positive Psychology and Lifestyle

"Keep yourself positive and alive both inside and outside."

One of the most important things I learned while dealing with cancer is to keep myself alive during the journey. Don't die before you actually die. Keep your spirit high and give your best as if you are playing in the World Cup finals. Watch many inspirational videos, read books, take up a sport if you wish, watch entertaining shows, be with nature, observe what is going inside, dive deep within and introspect on life and its purpose, connect with the self, and pamper yourself sometimes. I preferred the company of people who wanted to be with me non-judgmentally. I did not mind people with favorable judgments though! I liked those who said I looked well. I liked those who said I looked happy. I did not want to spend time with those who asked me if I had lost weight, especially if I had not lost weight. I did not like to be with people asking if 'I have done all the tests to make sure the cancer is not back.' I did not like people asking me 'if I am cancer-free.' I preferred to wear nice clothes to look healthy to myself and others. Some comments sound like the person needed proof that the cancer was not back. Some comments sound as though they think that there is cancer until proven otherwise. Some other comments sound as though they are surprised that I am doing well. All these people mean well but do not know what to ask. I have to admit that some comments hurt. It feels as though the person pulls me down when I am trying to stay afloat. Sometimes, the difference between living in 'Infinity' and living in 'uncertainty' is minimal. But we, the cancer survivors, are a different breed. We like to live in our own blissful world with unconditional joy. We do everything to get rid of cancer, go for tests to monitor our health, and like to live 'cancer-free.' We don't want additional proof that there is no cancer. We undergo tests to make sure that we are cancer-free. We look for the 'presence of healthy tissues' and not the 'absence of cancer'! Even though they mean somewhat the same, they play differently in our minds. We like to deal with cancer in such a way as to be in 'Infinity.'

xiii. Stay away from too many gadgets!

In this era of an abundance of social media, it is easy to spend several hours every day with our smartphones, iPads, tablets, and computers. This takes away your time from family, reading, listening, planning, and contemplation. As there is a lot of exposure to unknown radiation, it is a good habit to stay away from radiation in any form as much as possible. Keep your gadgets away as much as possible and be with nature. It is a good idea to put a limit on daily screen time and schedule 'no gadget' time when you don't use the gadgets. The new phones monitor your screen time and allow you to monitor it. It is up to you to decide how much screen time is reasonable for you. But I suggest limiting non-work/school-related screen time to three hours a day. My friend, Sunil Tulsiani, suggests not using electronic gadgets for two hours before bed. He also recommends not charging any computers and cell phones close to your bedroom when sleeping. Robin Sharma, of 'Monk Who Sold My Ferrari?' fame, recommends longer 'no gadget time' in his book, '5 AM Club'. Tony Robbins also recommends no gadgets for two hours before going to bed. Proximity to fresh air, water, and earth probably heals the body much faster than limiting yourself to a room and a few gadgets.

There was a paper in the New England Journal of Medicine showing a higher risk of a brain tumor in cell phone users. This paper emerged when cell phone use was not as rampant as today. In this day and age, everyone is a cell phone user. I have a dentist friend who does not carry a cell phone even in 2022! But there aren't many such people in this world. Some people use headphones with or without Bluetooth. I guess they reduce the 'exposure' to whatever toxic waves the cell phones emit. Some companies sell certain chips that you apply to the back of your phone to reduce the 'toxic wave' exposure to your body. I called it a 'toxic wave' because I am unsure if these are electromagnetic radiation, inaudible sound waves, or other unknown things. This is not mainstream practice, so many would call these practices scams. I am not an expert in this field and, hence, cannot make recommendations. But I use a chip I paid 100 US$ for and bought from a random Swedish person whom I met in a non-medical meeting. I was not convinced enough to spend 400 US$ to buy a chip for my wife and children, and I was not convinced enough to ask all my other family members and friends to buy it. I consider myself at higher risk of developing cancer than people who have never had cancer, and for that reason, sometimes I do some random, unproven things. I suggest setting a limit on your screen time or assigning a no-screen time in your day. Other things are optional.

xiv. Accept, fight, and be the witness to your body, mind, and intellect

'Great things come from HARD WORK & PERSEVERANCE, no excuses.'

Kobe Bryant

More on positive psychology! I changed my attitude from panicking to complete acceptance and fighting the challenge with serenity. The moment I accepted it as a challenge and a game, I got the inner strength to give my best to play every move. I also made sure to answer everyone's concerns and questions. Study the non-dualistic philosophy (called 'Advaita' in Sanskrit from Eastern Indian Hindu Philosophy) or the power of 'Now' by Eckhart

Tolle. You will learn to witness what is going on in your body and not be part of it. You are the witness to your body, your emotions, and your intellect. You are your light of lights. You are the 'NOW' that Eckhart Tolle talks about. The real you are the infinite consciousness within you. You are that 'Infinity' in you. You are the 'ONE' within you. You are that fearless, enemy-less, birthless, deathless, dimensionless, attributeless blessing and spark within you. You are 'THAT'. You are 'Infinity'. This is positive psychology that is being taught in leadership classes these days.

This Infinity is referred to in the sports world as well. Referring to the legendary soccer player Leonel Messi from Argentina, who wears the number 10 jersey, Cirque creative director Sean McKeown says, "to find the ten that we all have inside." Guess what! Argentina and Leonel Messi won the COPA soccer cup again in 2024! Legendary cricket player Sachin Tendulkar is referred to as "the God of cricket," referring to the manifestation of Infinity in his cricket skills. Similarly, other legends like Michael Jordan, Roger Federer, Serena Williams, Tom Brady, and others in various fields are referred to by similar superlatives. Depending on how you connect with it, you can consider it as religious, spiritual, or scientific inner engineering. Some call it religious and spiritual, some call it spiritual but not religious, and some call it neither religious nor spiritual. Some call it scientific technology, positive psychology, or inner engineering. All of them are true and relevant.

Since cancer affects my body and I am not this body, cancer has affected my body. Cancer has not affected me. I can, hence, disown cancer and witness it disappearing in front of me. I like to witness it as a witness and not be the one with cancer.

xv. Transform lifestyle

Once you are diagnosed with cancer, it is essential to transform your lifestyle. I embraced many changes, from changing my diet to practicing deep meditation. These mainly included food, sleep, exercise, meditation, connection with self, and much more. A detailed explanation of this is described later in this book. The prayer, 'Lead me from untruth to truth, darkness to light, and mortality to immortality,' is very relevant and practical to meditate upon 24/7.

xvi. Saying the right things and not saying the wrong things, more on positive psychology

Friends and family were the most potent sources of strength during my cancer. They uplifted and motivated me to do my best. I am blessed with a highly caring group of friends who were there with me throughout the journey. My family did not lose hope, and that gave me the strength to fight the unbearable pain of cancer.

Some patients assign one person the responsibility of communicating with friends and family through phone calls, social media, and blogs. I did not do that. However, since social media technology has changed since then, I would make a private Facebook page, a private blog page, or a WhatsApp group in this day and age. I took all the phone calls because I wanted to. Some people filter the calls, and I did not want to do it. In 2004, 'caller ID' was a subscribed item in phones, and we used to get fewer unsolicited phone calls. I wanted to be reachable to my family and friends who cared for me. I had no enemies, and I have none today. I am not a celebrity and I only got enough calls that I could handle myself. I knew it was hard for me to explain to people repeatedly. Indeed it was. But I owed it to them. The first few weeks were difficult for me to explain the same thing so many times to multiple friends and family members. Many well-meaning people don't know what to tell a friend with cancer and end up saying things you don't want to hear. Some of the statements I don't want to hear are: 'You have lost weight,' 'You look weak,' 'You look sick,' 'I am sorry for you,' 'Who will take care of your children,' 'How did you get cancer?', 'Don't worry! Some miracle will save you,' 'You would not have got this if you had done or not done something' and many others. Sometimes, I had to educate people on what to say. Sometimes, I had to avoid situations that would initiate such discussions. But I have also had people I barely knew call me and offer help or give encouraging words. I enjoyed most of these calls and still remember many of them.

There are a few ways friends can support the patient's family by motivating them to thrive through this journey instead of saying unpleasant words even out of concern. What we tell has a lot of power and influence. Hence, we have to exhibit that responsibility when we communicate. I listened to this impressive keynote address by Rachel Callander during the Annual Dialysis Conference 2022, and I realized that my examples also fall into four quadrants with different names. She was talking about communicating with parents and children in the healthcare field.

Figure: Impact of what and how we tell people with cancer (Inspired by Rachel Callander)

Good EMPOWERING examples of what you should say are:

- You look great

- You look wonderful

- You look well

- You look happy

- Your eyes look bright

- I heard you are doing great

- I learn from you

- I feel better talking to you

- You are the sun that oozes positive energy and light

- You have sun on your face; you make people smile

- I look better standing next to you

- Nice shirt/dresses/pants/shoes/belt/tie/socks

- Nice necklace

- You have a wonderful smile ('Smile takes you an extra mile' according to my friend Dr. Raju)

- You make others better

- Is something bothering you? You look preoccupied. Is there anything I can do for you?

- You have an 'Infinity'/infinite strength/unique spirit within you

- Some jokes /humor

Some examples of FLUFFY (encouraging, but not empowering) comments you may say are:

- You can do whatever you aspire for

- Everything is changing; this will also change

- Everything is momentary like Buddha says; suffering is also momentary

Some examples of ANNOYING things you can avoid are:

- You have lost hair

- Don't worry, some miracle will save you

- I am sorry for you.

- You have lost weight

- You have gained weight

Good DESTRUCTIVE examples of what you should not say are:

- Has your cancer spread?

- Which all body parts have cancer spread to?

- Are you sure that your cancer has not spread?

- You don't look well

- You look sick/unwell/weak

- You look older

- Your breath smells

- Did the doctor tell the prognosis?

- Did the doctor say how long you are going to live?

- Who is going to take care of your children?

- If you had prayed regularly and in such a way, you would not have developed cancer

- I have been telling you not to eat junk food and not to smoke. If you would have listened to me or your spouse, you would not have developed cancer.

- I did not think you would make it

- If you had not left your country, you would not have developed cancer

Finally, even when you say a good thing to somebody going through cancer, it is essential, to be honest to yourself in your heart. We, the 'cancer-people,' understand when you fake even though we like hearing good things. We like being loved, probably a little more than others. We don't like sympathy, but we love to be loved. Sometimes, we like to be hugged! We like some gentle assuring pat on our shoulders. We like you to look deep inside our eyes and say something nice and encouraging.

xvii. Financial planning, health insurance terminologies, and advanced care planning

I had three months to get chemotherapy and radiation and wait for the area to heal before having the big surgery. I explained to my wife about our finances and what she had to do if I were to die. I also invited my insurance agent to my home and had him explain to my wife what to do if I were to die. I showed her where the insurance policy is kept at home. It is a good idea to share the passwords with your spouse. Having a living will, advanced directives, and medical power of attorney is always a good idea. The best time to do this is when you are well. I already had a will. You do not need to hire an attorney to do advanced directives and medical power of attorney, even though I had an attorney do one for me. All you need is the appropriate paperwork that you can get from hospital social workers.

You can also get these documents online. You have to have two witnesses who are unrelated to you or one witness and a notary.

If you live in the United States, it is good to know the difference between 'copay' (what you pay at the time of seeing a doctor)' and 'deductible' that I learned after I became a patient myself. For example, you may have to pay nothing to your primary care doctor when you have an annual physical examination, $ 20$ when you see your primary care doctor for any other reason, and $ 50$ when you visit a specialist like an oncologist or surgeon. This is a 'co-pay'. You may have to pay 20% of the charges when you have a CT scan. This is the deductible. Once you spend a certain amount of money on co-pays and deductibles during the year, you get 100% coverage. For example, if your deductible is 2500$, once you spend 2500$ in deductibles and copays since the beginning of the year, you get full coverage and stop paying deductibles until the end of the year. The cycle repeats again the following year. If you know that you will be spending a lot during the following year, it is better to put the maximum allowable amount of money in a 'flexible spending account (FLEX)' or 'health saving account (HSA)', depending upon what your employer offers. In FLEX, you lose it if you don't spend it during that year. In HSA, you can spend the money at any time in the future. Some hospital staff might ask you if you have made your funeral arrangements! My wife was asked this question at some odd time when I was in the operating room! 'Indians' from the Indian subcontinent generally don't do funeral planning! I still have not done my funeral planning. But if you are comfortable with it, it is probably a good idea. In the US, it costs about 5000 to 10,000$ for cremation and more for burial. I know people who have made their funeral arrangements and have paid for such arrangements while they are alive to reduce the burden on the family after they die.

Cancer care and treatment are generally costly. Cancer not only takes a toll on your health, emotions, and time but on your finances too. It is best to be covered by a health insurance policy to fight any uncertainty visiting us unexpectedly. However, there may be unexpected charges which are not covered by the health insurance policy. When you are emotionally drained and physically weak, tracking finances creates more stress and takes your energy. In such a situation, relying on a family member or friend to keep track of costs for you is alright. Ask this person to go with you to doctor visits and help with all this planning. You can also discuss and take inputs from this person about the financials and how much more funds would be needed and to be prearranged.

Here are some tips for managing your financials well, some ideas on how to plan and discuss treatment costs with your healthcare team:

People with cancer have medical treatments, such as office visits, traveling costs, lab tests, imaging tests like MRI, CT scans, and X-rays, invasive procedures such as placement of ports for infusion of chemotherapy medicines, oral medicines, surgery, radiation treatments, hospital stays, home care set up if required, walkers, canes, wheelchairs, shower chairs, other durable medical equipment, special referrals, etc. Talk with your healthcare team and find answers to the questions related to you and your treatment.

How long will I need to be treated, and what is the estimated total cost of my proposed treatment plan? Are there any treatment options that might cost less, and how well will they work?

How much will my insurance pay for each of my treatment options, and how much will I have to pay myself?

Does my health insurance company need to pre-approve any part of the treatment before I start?

Is there any way I can get ? Who can I contact about financial assistance or help setting up a payment plan?

Where will I get treatment? In the hospital, office, or at home?

If you are taking chemotherapy, find out how much the prescription might cost and if your health care team knows of patient assistance plans that can help . Don't be disappointed if the doctor or the front office representative does not have answers to your financial questions. You may have to speak to someone in the billing department and sometimes call your insurance company.

Sometimes, oral chemotherapy and chemotherapy infusions are billed differently. For Medicare beneficiaries in the US, oral chemotherapy gets billed to Medicare D, and intravenous chemotherapy administered in the office gets billed to Medicare Part B. In some situations, getting chemotherapy as an infusion in the doctor's office may be better financially than getting oral treatment. Infusions given in the doctor's office may be cheaper than those administered in the hospital. In some situations, oral chemotherapy can be as effective as intravenous chemotherapy.

Find out from your healthcare team what other prescription drugs you may need along with your cancer treatment, such as drugs to prevent nausea, treat pain, help with anxiety or depression, or control diarrhea. You might call a few pharmacies to know where you can get the best price. Sometimes, using applications such as GoodRx will cost less than using the insurance card. Download the 'GoodRx' application to your phone and enter the name of the medicine to check the price yourself. This is my free advertisement for GoodRx! Other agencies offer this service too. Recently, Mark Cuban, a billionaire and the owner of my favorite basketball team (Dallas Mavericks), started an online pharmacy called 'Cost Plus Drug Company' offering generic medicines, including some chemotherapy medicines, at a deep discount. Thank you, @MCuban, for helping thousands of patients and thousands of sports fans! This works in the US. I don't know if this works outside the US. @MCuban, if you read my book, your honest book review at amazon.com will mean a lot to me and will help more people get my message of navigating cancer!

If you have to stay in the hospital for any treatment options, you can just find out if your insurance company needs to pre-certify any services that you will receive during your hospital stay.

Find out if you will need services such as rehabilitation or home health care or medical devices after you leave the hospital.

To ensure that the health insurance company pays the bulk of your expenses and you are not overloaded by too much cost, you should know the insurance policy terms. Be aware of preferred or network doctors, hospitals, and clinics in your area. Maintain the records of health care costs and all documents carefully. If your treatment might be done from somewhere else apart from network doctors and hospitals, know the cost involved in it from your insurance company.

Usually, health care facilities and treatment centers have a financial department that handles health insurance concerns and problems. Ask your health care team if someone can help you with claims that are sent to the insurance company. In case you are short of funds, friends and family can approach cancer funding organizations or raise funds collectively. Some people use online services such as 'gofundme' to seek funds from friends and even unknown sources.

(Source: Most of this information is extracted from the write-ups of the American Cancer Society. I have added some more information for your benefit including the names of GoodRx, Cost Plus Drug Company, and 'gofundme' even though it is not my endorsement.)

Chapter Four

Surgery And a Few Months After Surgery

I had the big surgery on February 3, 2005. My preparation started a few months before the surgery. Generally, radiation causes swelling all around the area that is irradiated and it increases the risk of bleeding and non-healing after the surgery. So I had to wait for six weeks after completing radiation. I had lost five to six pounds of weight during chemotherapy and radiation. I knew that I would lose more weight after surgery. At 145 pounds of body weight and 5 feet 8 inches in height, I did not need to lose weight. I wanted to gain at least five pounds of weight before surgery to give me some allowance to lose it after surgery. I ate well, drank some generic (Equate®) brand of Ensure Plus® most of the days, and gained some weight to be two to three pounds above my baseline weight. Eventually, after surgery, I ended up losing nineteen pounds of weight that I have gained since then.

i. Preoperative visit with the surgeon

Mentally, I was ready to get the whole thing called cancer taken out of my body. My surgeon, Dr. Skibber, had given me about a 50% chance of not having a permanent colostomy. During the initial visit, he had not given me a rosy prognosis. He had quoted about a 60% chance of being cancer-free at five years and had warned me that young people can sometimes have more aggressive cancer. I did not necessarily like hearing that. My brother Ashok's presence was a big emotional help for me during this process. I have observed him the most and spent the most time with him during my formative years among all my four siblings. I always looked up to him as a sign of strength and I still do. He was going to come with me to meet the surgeon before the surgery. I warned Ashok that Dr. Skibber can be brutally honest and truth sometimes is not pleasant to listen to. I had an MRI scan and blood draws before the visit. Contrary to my expectations, he was optimistic. He said that MRI showed that the tumor had shrunk and that most of cancer that is seen in the scan may be dead cancer cells. He also said that it was unlikely that my prostate was involved. He did not necessarily verbalize that the anal sphincter would be preserved, but the way he talked after proctoscopy (a little unpleasant office procedure where they look into the anal canal by inserting a four-inch-long rigid tube called proctoscope) sounded very optimistic that I would do well after surgery. It sort of meant to me that my anal sphincter would be preserved by all probability that I would not need a permanent colostomy and that I would well.

ii. Preoperative anesthesiology and cardiology visits

This was an interesting visit! I had already chosen the anesthesiologist suggested by my anesthesiologist sister from a different hospital in the same city, almost the same campus; they call it 'the Medical District', apparently the largest one in the world! But she mainly takes care of children. The reason for the pre-op visit is to make sure I am medically as fit as I can be for the surgery. In a planned surgery it is better to go for surgery in as fit a situation as possible. If you have lost weight and are underweight, it is better to gain back some of that weight before surgery. After surgery, you are likely to lose some weight. Being strong helps recover from the surgery faster. I lost 19 pounds (8.5 Kg) after surgery that I have gained back since.

In the preoperative visit generally, you don't get to see the same anesthesiologist who is going to take care of you in the operating room. All the blood test results were good. To make things interesting, my electrocardiogram (EKG or ECG) showed some abnormalities. I was impressed with the maturity of my preop anesthesiologist. I was intrigued with how laid back he was and in my mind, I disagreed with his comment about how useless physical examination was. I take pride in my history and physical examination. Most doctors all over the world do. Sir William Osler, M.D., often described as the father of modern medicine, told his students: "He who studies medicine without books sails an uncharted sea, but he who studies medicine without patients does not go to sea at all." Medical school faculty continue to teach such advice to their students today. Clinical observation has been a part of medicine since Indian, Egyptian, Babylonian, and Chinese physicians began examining the body thousands of years ago. Many of the doctors in the US do better history and physicals than anybody I know. Dr. Abraham Verghese, a Stanford medical professor born in India, trained in India, Ethiopia, and the US, who emphasizes the importance of physical examinations, has risen to fame from his speeches and book on physical examination. He says this about listening to the heart of a dying man: *I will never leave you. I will not let you die in pain or alone.* I took some of these lines from a New York Times article and from the website of Yale University. Needless to say, history and examination have their value in clinical medicine, but they have their limitations as well. They do not tell me how good my kidneys are. They do not tell you how extensive the cancer is unless it is very extensive with palpable liver and lymph nodes. Similarly, it may not tell an anesthesiologist about my perioperative risks.

He showed me the clinical practice guidelines by the American College of Cardiology on his smartphone and told me that asymptomatic EKG abnormalities don't need any different care since I did not have any cardiac symptoms. I think he showed me the guidelines because I am a physician. Nevertheless, I was impressed that he was not too excited about the EKG abnormality and he practiced evidence-based medicine. I was very satisfied with his compassionate, confident, mature, and knowledgeable approach. Moreover, I appreciated him for making me feel involved in my care.

But the curious 'me' was not satisfied enough. I got worried looking at my EKG. I knew that I was having major surgery and the complication rate is higher if I don't have a healthy heart. I thought that I might need heart catheterization before surgery to conclusively rule out blockages in the heart. What if I can't have surgery because of a heart problem? I would have been in deep trouble if I were to have a bad heart and cancer at the age of 41 years. Remember I was playing in the 'World cup finals'! There was no room for errors. I called my trusted cardiologist friend, Dr. Imran Afridi, in Dallas and faxed him my EKG. He was and still is the best non-invasive cardiologist I know in Dallas. He read the EKG and told me that I had a benign EKG abnormality (called repolarization changes), reassured me, and agreed to see me the very next day. The next day, he examined me, did a stress test, EKG and echocardiogram in Dallas, and cleared me for surgery. He did all this free of cost. We have this courtesy that people from the same profession don't charge fees to each other. Barbers don't charge barbers and doctors don't charge doctors! Sailors don't charge the 'God' because both the sailor and the God are in the same business of helping people cross the ocean of life with its waves of difficulties.

In the epic Ramayana, the boatman ('*Kevat*' in Hindi) did not accept a gift from God Rama (God who came to this earth as a human being) after he helped him cross the Yamuna river for the reason that both the boatman (rower) and God help people cross the river of life with its waves as difficulties. He reminded God that people from the same profession don't charge fees to each other. Sometimes accepting fees decreases the value of the help you received or offered. A word of caution is that in the US, I have been told that it is against the law to not collect the copay and bill the insurance for the remaining part of the fees. If you don't collect the copay, you cannot bill the insurance. Dr. Afridi did exactly that. More importantly, he provided medical care that was par excellence. It may sound strange to many, but health insurance companies have a lot of clout in politics and law in the US.

Being a physician helped me get things done quickly. It may or may not matter medically, but it helped me manage my life efficiently. For the non-physician readers, please be assured that I take excellent care of my patients whether I know them personally or not. You are like my family once I see you. Most physicians are like me. You don't need to know the doctors to get excellent medical care.

iii. Mental preparation for surgery and some hiccups before the surgery

I took my brother and my mother-in-law who had also come from India to help us to my sister's house in Houston before the surgery. Gopal Ponangi, a good friend, called me on my way to Houston and I told him that I would like to go for surgery in a positive state of mind. I think I told him that I did not want anyone to get emotional and cry prior to the surgery.

When I was all set for surgery, I started feeling feverish the day before surgery with a sore throat. I took some antibiotics. It is not ideal to have an elective surgery with a respiratory tract infection. I also felt that if I let go of this operation date, I might not get OR (operating room) time soon enough. Moreover, my brother and mother-in-law had come from India for three weeks and if the surgery were to be postponed beyond three weeks, I felt that they would not be able to wait even though they did not say that. I was scared to inform my surgeon fearing that he may postpone the surgery. My sister assured me that children undergo surgeries when they have minor upper respiratory infections since they get infections all the time. As the day passed, I felt more and more uncomfortable and felt obliged to inform my surgeon. I gathered courage and called him at 5:20 p.m. He promptly replied that we should proceed with the surgery as long as I have no fever. He also said that the anesthesiologist will make a final decision in the morning when he checks on me before the surgery. My uncle, Dr. Sugandh Shetty, flew from Detroit. My good friends, Raju and Sumit, flew from Dallas and we all gathered at my sister's house. We all sang some Hindu devotional songs and my sister's babysitter originally from Nigeria sang a Christian prayer. I slept well and woke up fresh. We all prayed again, I recited *Gayatri Mantra* 108 times and we went to the hospital in a positive state of mind. The *Gayatri Mantra* is considered a very powerful mantra and we played it non-stop in my hospital room 24 hours a day, every day after my surgery. Everybody was tense and calm at the same time, and nobody cried. Remember, I did not want anybody to cry and wanted to go to surgery in a positive state of mind! That was a perfect integration of science, positive psychology and spirituality in cancer care.

iv. Pain management

Doing a pain-free surgery is the basic requirement for any surgery. Anesthesiology is a very precise science that only they know better. In addition to putting you to sleep, for big surgeries, they also do epidural anesthesia to manage pain after surgery. This involves an expert doctor placing a small flexible tube (catheter) in the space just outside the spinal cord. Medicine is constantly infused to numb the nerves as they leave the spinal cord. My sister made sure that this epidural catheter was placed by a skilled doctor and not a trainee. She was also playing the 'World Cup Finals' game with me. The senior physician was pleasant and did the procedure uneventfully. I am told that there are other options to manage post-operative pain now; one of them that intrigued me is injecting some long-acting pain medicine at the site of surgery at the time of surgery. This is done by the surgeon.

After having the epidural catheter inserted in the pre-op area, the next thing I knew was that I woke up in the recovery room after surgery. This is the room where patients get monitored after surgery. Dr. Skibber, my surgeon said that he was able to save the sphincter and was able to remove cancer till the margins were cancer-free. This is something that they check before closing the wound.

During the surgery, I of course did not know what was going on. Later I found out that my brother, Ashok was 'caught' crying while I was being wheeled to the OR. He was hiding his emotions from me because he had heard me say that I did not want anyone to cry. Thank you, *anna,* for your help and I am sorry that I may have 'forced' you to not express your emotions in front of me. Apparently, everyone was tense while I was undergoing surgery. Two people were God-sent to keep my family members calm and occupied. One was a volunteer and she visited me before I left the hospital at our request. I don't remember her name. She was a Caucasian female probably in her 40's. She was a beautiful soul in all ways, extremely pleasant, loving, compassionate, sophisticated, and very positive. I and my family members feel indebted to her. Volunteers are a big part of the functioning of US hospitals. They contribute thousands of hours to the hospitals. Another God-sent person was Dr. Ruben Velez, my boss and the President and CEO of Dallas Nephrology Associates (DNA) at that time. He apparently reduced a lot of stress with his humor. My brother, my sister, and my brother-in-law are very grateful to him and they always talk about him. I may not have thanked him enough, but I am very grateful to him for the many ways he helped me. Apparently, when my family members thanked him profusely, he told them that he does not have to be thanked since he is part of our family and I am part of his family. That is the greatness of DNA and I know that we in DNA are one big family. On a lighter note, he hooked me for life. I could never think of leaving DNA or him since then and I am not planning to.

Incidentally, another strange thing had happened when I was in the operating room. My wife was told that she had a phone call from the social services department. When she picked up the phone, one lady asked her, 'Madam, has Mr. Shetty arranged for his funeral?'. My wife was shocked. What would anybody feel? Her husband is in surgery and someone calls to ask her about funeral arrangements! She told her that she did not know about it. After that, the person told her that this is just a formality. Indeed, it is a very cruel formality! It is possible that somebody forgot to ask that question before my surgery. Somebody forgot to cross some 'T's and was trying to save her job! This was not positive psychology!

The first person among my 'family' members that I saw after I woke up from surgery was Dr. Velez. I was surprised because I was expecting my wife or my sister to visit me first. But he somehow managed to see me before he could come back to Dallas and report to my DNA family. After that Mala, Shakku, Ashok and others visited me by turns.

Initially, my pain control was good. One of the side effects of epidural analgesia is that it can drop your blood pressure. My blood pressure dropped too and the doctors had to make a difficult decision of stopping epidural analgesia to bring the blood pressure up. My pain knew no end! After having major surgery in my belly and the bottom (anal area), I was getting no pain medicines! My sister Shakku, after unsuccessful negotiation with my nurse, spoke to the pain service anesthesiologist and managed to get an order for a small dose of pain shot. It was a big relief getting that order, but the few minutes that it took to get the medicine from the pharmacy felt like an eternity while I was writhing in pain. I know that if Shakku was not there with me, I would have suffered from pain much longer. They eventually did give me a gentle dose of injectable pain medicine. Remember that injectable pain medicines can also drop your blood pressure. If the blood pressure drops too low for a prolonged period of time, you can die. So the doctors and patients are in between a rock and hard place. If you decide to be safe and hold the pain medicines because the blood pressure is too low, the patient has to suffer more pain. But if you decide to give pain medicine to relieve the pain when the blood pressure is low, it can be unsafe to the patient's life. Doctors always will choose to have a live patient with pain than a dead patient with no pain! You are damned if you do, damned if you don't! This is the challenge of pain medicine.

Doctors who treat pain can be blamed no matter what they do. If you give enough pain medicine to relieve pain, you are blamed for giving medicine that has a tendency for dependency and causing constipation. If you give too little medicine, you are blamed for not controlling the pain adequately. But it was a very painful experience for me when they stopped the epidural analgesia. The few minutes that nurses took to get the pain medicine injection appeared like an era! Those were frustrating times when I wished that a person such as the 'pain management nurse' physically went to the pharmacy to procure the medicine right away. But that is not how the system works. Once the order is placed in the computer, the pharmacist has to dispense the medicine after which the pharmacy technician brings the medicine to the nurse from the pharmacy. The time taken would depend upon the time taken by the pharmacist to dispense the medicine and the time taken by the technician to bring the medicine from the pharmacy to the ward/the floor that the patient is in and the time taken by the nurse to find the medicine and administer it to you, the patient. All these three people use their priorities to work on your case. For you, the patient, there is only one priority, your pain and there is only one patient, you! But for the pharmacist, the pharmacy technician, and the nurse, there are other patients too. Some of them may be sicker than you, some of them may be in more pain, some of them may be more demanding, and some of them may be nicer than others. Every little thing matters when human beings are involved. After all, we are emotional animals. In pain management, the medical system has a system to reduce the number of steps to efficiently deliver the medicine and also to keep accountability of people handling these medicines which can be abused. Some medical units keep the pain medicines readily available to the nurses without having to go to the pharmacy. When you are in pain, every second is too long till you get pain relief. Every second of pain is too many seconds with pain.

I may not have been very nice to my nurses at that time of extreme pain and if that was the case, I apologize to the nurses who took care of me. Some efficiency in this area could reduce the amount of pain. It would have been better if a clinician assessed me at that time and decided to administer more fluids to bring up my blood pressure in a more timely fashion so my pain could have been managed more efficiently. This is for the pain management doctors to note if you have taken a commitment to manage pain. But please know that determination of the need for fluids in the evaluation of low blood pressure is very difficult, even for doctors. I remember my professor and Director of Nephrology, Dr. Karl Skorecki at the University of Toronto telling me once that I would win the Nobel prize if I came up with a method to accurately determine this. Twenty-eight years later, we haven't still solved that puzzle. But there is some inefficiency built into any system and every system! The medical system is no exception. I saw my sister cry and apologize to me when she could not help my pain even though she is an anesthesiologist herself. My heart rate was very fast and they had to call a cardiologist who determined that my heart was good and I needed more intravenous fluids. It helped bring my blood pressure up so I could get adequate doses of pain medicine.

Pain management during the subsequent days after surgery is also tricky, especially after operating on your belly. On one hand, you need good pain relief and on the other hand, you don't want to slow down the intestinal contractions and bowel movements. I had slow bowel movements after surgery; it is called 'paralytic ileus' in medical language. Here the intestine slows down, there will be no bowel movements, there will be no flatus passing down, belly distends and it hurts. It hurts a lot sometimes and you cannot eat or drink anything till the bowel moves. Sometimes they have to introduce a nasogastric tube in your nose that goes to your stomach to relieve the distention. They did that to me and it helped reduce the pain. Insertion of that tube (called nasogastric tube) was not that uncomfortable.

Passing flatus and feeling hungry are generally good signs suggesting your way to recovery. When that happens, the tube will be removed. It can take a few days to weeks to recover. Most recover in a week. Once you get good bowel movements and once the pain is better and you tolerate food, you get to go home. I was initially better after two days and was allowed to drink clear liquids. But then I developed pneumonia and 'paralytic ileus' requiring me to stay for a total of nine days in the hospital.

When you have 'paralytic ileus', pain management is tricky because if you take more pain medicine the recovery from 'paralytic ileus' can be delayed since the pain medicines (narcotics) slow down the intestinal movements ('peristalsis' in medical language). If you take less medicine, you don't get sufficient pain relief. It is common for you to be on PCA (patient-controlled analgesia) after surgery to allow patients to deliver additional doses of pain medicines within the safe limits that are set by your doctors. I was on PCA since I did not tolerate epidural analgesia and looking back, I felt that I took less pain medicine hoping to recover from 'paralytic ileus' faster. In this situation, you are damned in both ways you go. Another situation of tongue caught between your teeth! Generally, doctors like to relieve pain adequately in such situations. Those of you who have taken hydrocodone or codeine might remember getting constipated!

I have a little story here. Remember, I said I got worse on the third day after surgery. I developed bloating of the belly, pain, and fever. I was in a lot of pain. I was taken to radiology to get an X-ray of my chest to look for pneumonia. I was on PCA, patient-controlled analgesia. That means I was supposed to be in control of administering additional doses of pain medicines if I needed them. I was really in pain, a lot of pain, I was weak and frustrated. I was supposed to stand for the X-ray. But I was in pain and I was weak, it was going to be difficult to stand. The hospital staff who wheeled me in the wheelchair pushed the PCA pump's button so I could get an additional dose of the pain medicine before I stood to have the X-ray. The frustrated me did not appreciate her taking control of my PCA! I questioned her as to why she pushed the button. She replied very assertively and told me unapologetically, 'I have experienced pain before and I knew you were in pain, I did not want you to be in pain'. Even though she was wrong, I knew she was trying to help me and she was right! I just kept quiet. Moreover, she was so assertive that I did not have the strength to argue. I don't remember her name, she was a young African American lady. I thank her for feeling my pain and her contribution to reducing my pain. But control is so important, especially when you have no control over a lot of things in life. When you are sinking, you hang on to even little straws for support.

v. Colostomy or no Colostomy?

A colostomy is a procedure where the colon is opened to the skin surface in the left lower part of your belly. It is done in cancer of the lower part of the rectum where the risk of permanent incontinence is very high. In those who have a colostomy, the stool comes to a plastic pouch that generally is emptied every day. I was told that my cancer was fairly low and I had a high chance of needing a colostomy.

My surgeon, Dr. Skibber, at MD Anderson cancer center is specialized in preserving anal sphincter and avoiding colostomy and they have a world-famous nurse practitioner who has designed a bowel management protocol to reduce incontinence. Even though many patients live with colostomy without complaining and move on with their lives, it is nicer not to have it. My Oncologist Dr. Ajani strongly suggested that not having a colostomy will give me a better quality of life and I agree with him. I had a temporary ileostomy for about six months after surgery to allow the rectum to heal where they removed my cancer and part of the colon.

In 'ileostomy', the terminal small intestine is brought out to the skin surface on the right lower part of the abdomen and is attached to a plastic ileostomy pouch. I did not mind it, but I did not like it either. There is nothing to like in wearing a plastic pouch, sometimes filled with feces, on your belly! Ileostomy needs to be emptied more often than colostomy. I had a constant fear that it would leak. It indeed happened a few times, but not very often. It happened less than once in two months. I used to always feel a fecal smell even though my family members and friends said that I was not smelling. They make ileostomy bags with some charcoal in them to reduce the smell. Moreover, the ileostomy was on my beltline and I had to wear pants with a high waistline to avoid the belt rub on the mouth of the pouch. I sometimes considered wearing suspenders instead of belts, but I did not. I did not want to look much different than before. If I were to need a permanent colostomy, I probably would have considered wearing suspenders.

If I have to suggest something, I would recommend avoiding colostomy, but the priority is to get cancer out completely. In the big scheme of things, I don't think it is anybody's fault to have a colostomy. But I am living an incontinent life without colostomy and I have figured out a way to have 'continence' despite being incontinent. Please look for a dedicated chapter in this book and maybe another dedicated book addressing the details in the future. I would not recommend colostomy even if the chance of becoming incontinent is 100%.

vi. Managing fecal incontinence

It is not fun being incontinent. It is very humbling and intimidating to be incontinent. That feeling of being unable to control something that you had control over throughout your adult life is very humbling. It is hard to keep it a secret among the family and friends you go out with. Traveling becomes challenging. I tried the following regimen involving taking Imodium two tablets once or twice a day, six capsules or one teaspoonful of psyllium powder (Metamucil® is the usual brand, but generic versions are cheaper and equally good, in India it is called *isabgol*) with two ounces of water after each meal and no other fluids with meals and for one hour after meals. This program was based on recommendations from MD Anderson cancer hospital. It had some success till I got partial intestinal obstruction after five years of following it. It also gave a lot of pain in the belly because the main component of the success of this program was to keep the stools hard and I got spasmodic/colicky pain as the colon was trying to move the hard stools. I also tried Kegel's exercise, biofeedback, yoga and meditation, homeopathic medicine, and whatever I could think of. Nothing worked to make me continent enough even though all of them have helped me to some extent. They may also have helped me face incontinence better. I appreciate my child, Krishna who recognized once that I was pleasant and smiling even when I was totally out of control with my bowel movements in a shopping mall. I have had situations where I have had to go to the toilet five to six times an hour in public places such as restaurants. It happens more often when I visit India, probably because I tend to eat more there and lose control of what I eat when I am there. But incontinence did not stop me, it never did!

After I got an episode of partial intestinal obstruction requiring me to prepare for another major surgery, a surgeon colleague of my sister suggested that I try an enema to prevent the obstruction. Thank you Dr. Bailey from Methodist Hospital, Houston. Eureka! Daily enema or colon irrigation with about 1 – 1.5 liter of tap water at room temperature (NEVER PUT WARM WATER IN YOUR COLON AND DON'T PUT SOAP WATER IN YOUR COLON EVERY DAY) worked wonders for me. It emptied my colon so I did not have any fecal matter in my colon to have a fecal bowel movement for another 24 hours. So I did not have to go to the bathroom multiple times during the day in between seeing patients.

It miraculously relieved the pain in the belly that I had suffered for a few years. And, finally, I could drink as much fluid as I wanted at any time of the day or night without fearing fecal incontinence. I could urinate standing without the fear of having an accidental bowel movement! Small things mean a lot when you lose them. It takes about 90 minutes in the morning to irrigate my large intestine without risking accidents (involuntary bowel movements) later. My recommendation (not prescription) to incontinent people is to try daily colon irrigation/enema with 1 – 1.5 liter of tap water at room temperature every day after you get approval from your doctor. It has worked great for me and it might work for you as well. I have been doing it six to seven days a week for the last nine to ten years with great results. A word of caution, never use warm or hot water for enema/colon irrigation. More details of managing incontinence are described in the dedicated chapter later in the book.

vii. Proselytization in the hospitals

Many times, I thought of not writing this chapter to avoid becoming controversial. But I decided to keep it to bring up this issue of social injustice. It does not affect most parts of the western world. It is largely a problem affecting those belonging to the Hindu faith. I have very good friends from all faiths. I am a Hindu, but my best friend in school was a Catholic. I studied in Catholic schools. I was treated by a Christian oncologist, a Muslim oncologist, a Hindu oncologist, a Jewish surgeon, a Jewish Radiation Oncologist and two Muslim cardiologists. Doctors, nurses, dieticians, respiratory therapists of all different faiths of the world have been my health care providers and I am grateful to them. Faith is a personal thing. I have been taught that different faiths of the world offer different ways of reaching the same ONE God, one 'Truth', and that all these paths are valid. Large parts of the world from all the faiths honor this. But there is some 'organized system' in the world that does not honor other faiths. I call proselytization an 'organized system' because it is not done randomly by random people. It is very organized and in some parts of the world, it is an industry, a business. People get compensated for converting people's faith.

"Truth is one, but the wise men know it as many; God is one, but we can approach Him in many ways."

I have to share my painful experience with a missionary who unsuccessfully tried to change my faith while I was in the hospital. Indians are probably the most affected by proselytization in the history of mankind. India was ruled by Muslim kings from the middle-east and the Christian viceroys of the United Kingdom for about 800 years. During this time thousands of temples were looted and destroyed. A lot of wealth was looted from India. The GDP of India came down from around 10% to less than 1% of the world's GDP during these 800 years. Millions of Hindus were forced to change their faith, many were raped or killed. Since the independence of India in 1947, forcible conversion has gone down. But the conversion by coercion and by approaching the vulnerable people has increased. I thought this happened only in India. But when I was admitted to the hospital, I was in a lot of pain and was getting narcotics for pain control. I was told that I was a little bit confused due to having an infection and getting narcotics. But I remember being in a lot of pain and I also remember arguing something with my sister. My family probably was panicking. One missionary saw my worried brother outside my room. She asked him if we would like her to pray for me. He readily agreed. I have always appreciated people praying for me and I am grateful to them. I know that many of my patients and friends have prayed for me in the churches and temples in Dallas. After she came to my room I agreed for

her to pray for me, but I told her that I am a Hindu and I am fine being a
Hindu. I think I must have sensed what was coming. There she starts! She
went on ranting how she did not come to my room on her own and that
she was sent by Jesus. I was fine with that. Then to my astonishment, she
kept repeating, 'this is the time to change your faith'. More surprisingly, my
nurse was in the room and she participated in the 'prayer' and 'chanting'.
I was not alright with this. I felt encroached and more. I felt that my faith
was questioned at a very vulnerable time in my life. I felt that I was taken
advantage of. I reported to the Pastoral department of the hospital and
they agreed that it was wrong on the part of the missionary to approach
me to change my faith. They also reminded me that the missionary was not
a hospital staff and was just a visitor and that they have seen this happen
in the past. When the missionary called me back after two-three days to
see if we wanted her back in my room we told her that there was no such
need. Missionaries do a lot of good services when there is a crisis. But in
return, many of them ask the victims of the crisis to change their faith.
Whenever you help a vulnerable person and expect something in return,
it no longer becomes a service. It becomes a deal! When you do this to a
vulnerable person, it is disrespectful and it is an abuse of the vulnerable, a
social injustice.

The Song of God (Bhagavad Gita), the sacred book of Hindus explains
three kinds of 'charity', one expecting nothing in return, one for fame, and
one for something in return. Proselytization falls in the third category, the
most inferior among the charities. I feel that this is an insult to God. I
think that this is an insult to even Jesus Christ. I have not read the Holy
Bible fully, but I highly doubt Jesus Christ suggested this. I think that this
is a misinterpretation of the teachings of spreading love from the Holy
Bible. If anybody believes that they have a better God, they are limiting
the scope of God. If God indeed exists, there can be only one God for all

living beings of all faiths of the world. God is omnipotent and omniscient. Just like all rivers join the same ocean, different faiths have different ways and paths to reach the same God. If any faith claims exclusivity to God, I consider them ignorant. I can disregard someone else's ignorance. At least that is what some of my good friends suggested. I have been told that I am overreacting to this incident. I don't think I am overreacting. In fact, I think that I have not done enough. I continue to reject and condemn this social injustice to thousands of vulnerable people across the world. I have moved on. But that does not take away the social injustice that is happening to thousands of vulnerable patients across the world who are being abused in the name of religious freedom. I still don't appreciate it after so many years. I did not appreciate that the hospital did not take ownership of the problem even though it is true that these missionaries are not hospital employees. Anything that happens within the hospital building should be the hospital's problem. I had a meeting with the head of the Pastoral department, but it did not go too far. Some appropriately call this 'predatory proselytization' because these predators are waiting in the hospitals and refugee camps to invite their victims when they are most vulnerable.

My message to all the cancer patients of the world is that you did not develop cancer because you don't worship God, it is not because you did not worship God the right way, it is not because your God is not as good as someone else's God, it is not because you do not belong to a particular faith, it is not because God is upset with you, it is not because God is punishing you. There cannot be a disciplinarian God and God is not a 'punishing body'. You do not get cured just because you changed your faith. In a Christian majority country such as the US, most cancer victims are Christians. In Hindu majority countries such as India, most cancer victims are Hindus. In Saudi Arabia, most cancer victims are Muslims, and in Israel, most cancer victims would be Jews. If someone tells you that his/her God is better than yours, I feel sorry for his/her ignorance. You don't have to be God-fearing; you just have to be God-loving.

I am going to quote part of **Swami Vivekananda's speech at the World Parliament of Religions 1893 in Chicago** in which he recognized this problem of leaders of one religion claiming superiority over the other. He said, *"Brothers and Sisters of America, much has been said of the common ground of religious unity. I am not going just now to venture my own theory. But if anyone here hopes that this unity will come by the triumph of any one of the religions and the destruction of the others, to him I say, 'Brother, yours is an impossible hope.' Do I wish that the Christian would become Hindu? God forbid. Do I wish that the Hindu or Buddhist would become Christian? God forbid. It has proved to the world that holiness, purity, and charity are not the exclusive possessions of any church in the world and that every system has produced men and women of the most exalted character. In the face of this evidence, if anybody dreams of the exclusive survival of his own religion and the destruction of the others, I pity him from the bottom of my heart, and point out to him that upon the banner of every religion will soon be written in spite of resistance: 'Help and not fight', 'Assimilation and not Destruction', 'Harmony and Peace, and not Dissension."*

The proselytization industry has only gotten bigger and richer since then. The recently released movie, *The Kashmir Files*, shows another criminal version of proselytization in Kashmir, India.

More needs to be done about this social injustice. I, unfortunately, have not done enough to stop this or expose this to the public. I should have. One problem is that those who have not gone through this don't get it. I could not even convince some of my family members that this is a serious problem. Missionaries claim that they are advocating religious freedom.

My problem is that, why are you doing it on these vulnerable people at a vulnerable time?

I also want to quote from the scriptures that is self-explanatory and relevant here:

"There is only one God, not the second; not at all, not at all, not in the least bit."

(*Ekameva adviteeya Brahma...*from *Chāndogya Upaniṣad* 6.2.1)

"Supreme God (Brahman) itself is real, non-dual, extremely pure, the essence of knowledge absolute, taintless, supremely peaceful, without beginning or end, beyond all activity, always of the nature of bliss absolute, transcending all diversities created by illusion, eternal, the essence of joy, indivisible, immeasurable, formless, unmanifest, nameless, immutable, and self-effulgent".

(Vivekachoodamani, Verse 237 and 238)

viii. Unconditional love and support

"Warmth can be felt in the tone of our voice, the sincerity of our gaze, and the serenity of our actions." – *John McGee.*

Getting unconditional love is a blessing. This is more stuff on positive psychology in cancer care. To be able to love unconditionally means loving the person without expecting anything in return. In this situation, the player is looking for a lot of love, prayers, and healing energy. A lot of times, friends and family get confused about what to do and what not to do. They want to help and love the person but they don't know how they can really help the main player.

Here are a few tips to express your love and help.

- Send an encouraging mail every fortnight or once a month.

- Send funny text messages, GIFs or laughter shows that make the person laugh.

- Play some board games.

- Tell the person that you love him/her.

- Create a banner of encouraging messages. Family, friends, and colleagues can make an encouraging banner with lots of inspirational messages to keep the spirit high. My children and my sister's children drew beautiful cards with crayons and pencils conveying love in their own way. That was very precious.

- Drive him/her to doctor appointments, chemotherapy, and surgery: I was so blessed to have such wonderful family and friends to be there for me during my radiation, chemotherapy, and surgery. Thankfully, there were very few occasions when I needed help driving. It is a good idea to not drive if you are taking pain medicines that may make you sleepy or less alert. It is a good idea not to drive when you are in pain. I am guilty of driving when I was in pain after surgery and I may have passed red lights a couple of times. I am not proud of those instances. If one has soiled the clothes from an involuntary bowel movement, driving can become challenging due to the distracting inconvenience. I remember once after my CT scan in Houston, my brother-in-law, Suresh drove me back to Dallas, a four-hour drive. I had so much bowel movement in my diaper after drinking the dye for the CT scan that it spilled into my car seat. There was no way that I could have driven safely by myself in that mess. Thank you, Suresh, for being there for me, thick or thin!

- Fundraising: Cancer treatments are really expensive and might need additional funds. Friends and family can come together to raise funds and help financially. This is also a great way to show unconditional love. I was fortunate that my sister, Shakku, my brother-in-law, Suresh, and my mentor, Dr. Oreopoulos offered to help me financially. Thankfully, I did not need financial help, but it was good to know that help was available if I needed it. I also knew that I had other friends and family who would have helped me if I needed. Some people use online tools such as 'gofundme'. Please be sensitive to the family's emotions. Some patients may not appreciate you making their problem public. In those situations, you may have to seek funds without revealing the person's identity.

- Gift them something creative: Gifting them art therapy books, fiction/non-fiction books, diaries, or some creative items, which can help them to be lively is a good way to support them. Gift them books that narrate the story of survivors and how bravely and skillfully they survived. This will inspire them to fight and understand that they too can survive this battle. Don't give books about those who died of cancer no matter how interesting and inspiring it is for you. You can just give them any book that you think will keep them reading. Just staying busy itself is healing. Other gift items are flowers, music, movies, clothes, and others.

- Food: I have noticed that it is a common custom to send food to the family. Some like it and others don't find value in it. You can decide if it is appropriate for your friend or relative who just got diagnosed with cancer.

Too many gifts do not help and in my case, this had made me uncomfortable and upset. Too many gifts are sometimes a sign that the person who is gifting you is scared of losing you!

Chapter Five

After Cancer: Why Me? Introspection, Justification and Science

I. **Buddha's two arrows**

There is a Buddhist metaphor of the 'second arrow'. This metaphor of two arrows is relevant in any problem solving or response to a problem such as cancer. The first arrow refers to any problem that inevitably happens in life, cancer in my case. The first arrow is released without prior notice and it catches us unaware. The second arrow refers to our response to the first arrow. We have control over the second arrow and we should control it to favor us. The first arrow can be called destiny, but the second arrow is the destiny under your control. You can choose to be brave and face it, fight it, defeat it, run away from it depending upon the situation. You can complain about it and be miserable or choose to see what can be done to make life meaningful. You can complain, blame God, your situation, people around you, your insurance company, the politicians, your employers, and everybody and everything that you cannot control, or you can move on and do all the things that you can do to make the best out of what you have. You can choose to live a life filled with gratitude for what you have or you can choose an unhappy and bitter life. There is a saying, 'pain is inevitable, suffering is optional.' You can see the glass half full or half empty. I chose to see the glass always half full. I chose to see divinity in everything and everybody as I always say. When you do that you will only see good things in life. You will only see happiness in life. You can offer all your pain to God, and choose not to suffer. My Christian patients say always that Jesus Christ took all the pain from his pupils to himself. You can find references to this in scriptures from all the religions of the world. The Bhagavad Gita has put it in many different ways on many occasions.

ii. Why me? Why do things happen? Why do bad things happen to good people? Why not me?

Evil is relative. Evil is a human thing. We don't call a lion evil for eating a deer. We don't consider water evil after a flood. We don't consider earth evil after people die from earthquakes. We don't call fire evil after it burns a house. We don't consider a tree evil if the tree falls and hurts us. Why is there evil in this world if God is almighty and all-loving that we all believe? Why is there evil when everything is God-like as Vedanta (of Hinduism) states? Why did Adam eat the 'forbidden fruit' when he was told not to eat it? Why was he punished for eating the 'forbidden fruit' if he could not avoid eating it?

Why did I get cancer at the age of 41? Why did I get colorectal cancer when I never ate beef or pork? Why did my friend get colon cancer when he was a vegetarian all his life? I have been a compassionate doctor all my life. I have not hurt people or abused vulnerable people knowingly. If I have made mistakes, why did God not prevent me from doing them? In Hinduism, evil is considered to be ignorance. It believes that evil itself is ignorance. It believes that anything experienced is not me. It believes that everything seen is not me. When I experience something, what I experience is the object and I am the subject. When I have cancer, cancer is the object and I am the subject. The 'seen' and the 'seer' are different. The experience and 'experiencer' are different. The object and the subject are different. Awareness that the experiencer and the experienced are different is knowledge. This knowledge is 'enlightenment.'

This description is all good for intellectual discussion. But why did I get cancer? Why did I have so much suffering and pain? Did I? No! My body developed cancer, I did not! I did not suffer, my mind did! Really? Does that mean that all that I went through is unreal? Is my experience of going through surgery, pain, incontinence unreal? Was that not me? It is hard to convince my wife and children that I did not have cancer, it was just my body! There is no question that I experienced cancer and all the pain and suffering that went with it. The next level of understanding is that my body, my mind, my intellect, my soul, the God in me are all ONE. That means that my suffering is God's suffering. Should I be compassionate towards God because God is suffering? God does not need that. God is almighty, all-loving, all compassionate, and infinite. But it can be relieving that you can share the pain and suffering with God. You can transfer the burden on God and be relieved. We can be humble and transfer the burden of causation to that Infinite force. We can be humble and live with ignorance of the answer to the question, 'Why Me?'. All faiths struggle to answer this question. The Book of Genesis describes Adam and Eve eating the fruit from the forbidden tree of knowledge and evil and ends up getting cursed by God. One can question if God is almighty and fair, why did he not prevent Adam from eating the forbidden fruit? Does that mean that there is free will that is not controlled by God? Does that mean God does not control certain things? Does that mean certain unpleasant things happen and God does not prevent them?

Do we have free will? Is action pre-destined?

If God decides everything, what is my responsibility? Why is there evil/suffering if there is God? There are arguments for and against this. These arguments are from a YouTube video by Swami Sarvapriyananda.

His videos are very informative and I have learned a lot from him. My humble gratitude to him. Since I have added materials from other sources as well, please refer to his videos if you want to listen to his arguments directly.

The argument for free will

If I feel that there is free will, there is free will. When I do something, I feel that I have the choice to do what I want to do. Examples of free will are:

- Karma theory in eastern religions believes that you reap the consequences of your actions and sometimes the consequences show up in another birth. Here the action is an act of free will, but the consequences of an action are an argument against free will.

- Religions that believe in one life: According to the theory of justifying God, God gives some free will and if we misuse it, then we will be punished. Adam and Eve ate the forbidden fruit and they were punished.

The argument against free will

- Metaphysical and causal argument: Everything, every event, every act has a cause, known or unknown. If there is a cause, there has to be an effect. Similarly, if there is cancer, there has to be a cause, known or unknown. If the cause is unknown, my free will has no place.

- Religious/theistic argument: If God exists, and is omniscient, God already knows what decision I take, and then I don't have free will.

- Law of Karma: All Hindus, Buddhists, Jains and Sikhs believe in the law of Karma. Our past actions give rise to effects. In that case, my current decision is a mental event, predetermined, and hence is not free.

The Law of Karma is an argument for and against free will depending upon how you look at it!

Benjamin Libet experimented and found that those who raised the arm had electrical activities in the brain (EEG, electroencephalogram) way before the act (raising the arm) and before the decision was made. This modern neuroscience experiment showed that there is no free will. The decision was already predetermined. Once released from the barn, the horse is in charge, not me. Krishna says this multiple times in the Bhagavad Gita (3:27, 13:29; 14:19). God inside a person alone does all the work, an ignorant person with ego thinks (gets illusion) that he is doing. The one who says that I am Brahman (*Aham Brahmasmi*) realizes that 'I am the witness' to what goes on in the world and in my physical body. My body is a non-agent doer.

Rabbi Harold Kushner, in his book, "*When Bad things Happen to Good People*", tries to answer this question, 'Why Me'? He refers to his own son dying at an early age due to an incurable disease. He does not answer the question. He just comes with a suggestion or two to face the reality. *He says there is randomness in this world that nobody including God prevents.* The second suggestion he gives is that such random unfortunate events should not prompt people to lose faith in God, even though he suggests that we should drop the belief that God is omnipotent. He says that God has limitations. God is limited by the laws of nature, human nature, and human moral freedom. This is almost suggesting that 'Karma' can overrule God in my opinion!

Hinduism, Buddhism, Jainism, and Sikhism believe in Karma theory. In simple terms, Karma theory believes that we reap the fruits of our past actions and these actions could be from this birth or our previous births. People who believe that they have not done anything bad in this life can justify getting cancer by blaming that they may have done something bad in their previous lives to get punished in this life. Again this justifies something that cannot be proven. This does not still answer why God allowed me to do such things and later develop cancer. The non-dual philosophy of Hinduism also does not explain this differently except that it believes that everything including your body is God (Brahman). According to this belief, when I am suffering, God is also affected and hence God is also suffering. It just takes away part of the burden from me. In the early phase of the spiritual evolution of the person, according to non-dualism, the physical body simply is not 'me'. The real 'me' is just the Atma, which is also called the soul. This helps me disown my body and physical ailments and be a joyful soul by detaching myself from all that is finite and perishable including my own body and cancer affecting my body!

Another way of looking at life-changing events like cancer is that such events help us elevate our souls spiritually. Hence these experiences are opportunities for spiritual elevation and progress. The more luxuries we have, the more we are likely to forget God, and the more we are likely to be attached to material luxuries. In one of the Hindu texts called, *Srimad Bhagavatam*, the queen Kunti asks for a famous boon, "O Shree Krishna, please give me hardships, tribulations, and difficulties." Her explanation and reasoning for embracing miseries gave her opportunities to turn towards God than risk forgetting God.

There are cancer survivors who say that cancer was the best thing that happened to them and that they became better human beings after experiencing suffering. I would not go that far. Has cancer changed me for the better? Yes! Is that the best thing that happened to me? No way! Cancer is the worst thing that has happened to me and my family. I can disown it as much as I want. But I can still vividly see my 10 years old son cry with fear of losing his father.

Prof Huston Smith, the author of *The World's Religions* is known for not only studying but practicing Hinduism, Buddhism, Islam, and Sufism. Yet he continued to remain a Methodist Christian all his life. His beloved granddaughter was killed at a young age and he also witnessed his daughter die in front of him. Yet he whispered the same prayer to himself several times a day, "God, you are so good to me" in his relentless spirit of gratitude to God. The practice of gratitude regularly is a very powerful problem solver and stress reliever. I recommend that all of us practice gratitude every day, every moment. Some people write down three things that they are grateful for before going to bed. I have read that Sheryl Sandberg, Chief Operating Officer of Facebook, who lost her husband due to sudden death in her forties, does that and recommends that. You can repeat what you are grateful for. It can be as simple as being grateful for having food on the table. You can be grateful for having loving family or friends. You can be grateful to your compassionate nurse. You can be grateful to your husband. You can be grateful to your wife for everything she does. It is a good idea. Why not? A happy wife makes life happy. I cannot be grateful enough to my wife, children, family, and friends every day of my life.

More on why things happen

Arthur L. Herman in his book, 'The Problem of Evil and Indian Thought' identifies some 21 historical solutions to the problem of evil. 'This is a review of all the major arguments for why there is evil if there is a God who could prevent it and wants to. Beginning with the problem of evil in the West, Professor Herman traces the history of one of the most fascinating of all perennial philosophical puzzles. The author identifies some 21 historical solutions to the problem, which are then reduced to eight quite distinct solutions. Prof. Herman then turns in the second part of the book to the history of the problem of evil in Indian thought'. He starts with four premises: 'God is all-powerful, God is all-knowing, God is all good, and there is evil'. Then he asks "Why is there any misery at all in the world? Not by chance surely. Form some cause then. Is it from the intention of the diety? But he is perfectly benevolent. Is it contrary to his intention? But he is almighty. The author then joins the analysis of the problem of evil to the Indian doctrine of rebirth in order to attempt a solution to the problem. By careful analysis, the author shows that the doctrine of rebirth can satisfy the conditions already set forth as adequate for a solution to the problem of evil." This is the verbatim reproduction of a summary of Professor Herman's book from amazon.com and from his book.

Buddhism also addresses the question of why there is suffering. This quote summarizes it.

"Buddha: all compounded things decay. Everything is transitory in this world. Even pleasant things decay. Suffering is inevitable. Body, mind, and relationship will change."

According to the Buddhist perspective, the Buddha-nature ('Enlight-ened' nature') is the core of our being. In Buddha's later years, people came to him asking 'what' he was. Buddha answered, "I am awake (I am Buddha)". The next question to Buddha was: 'Is it male? Is it female?' and the answer was: 'All coming through in the sense of serenity—not just acceptance, but affirmation. It's a face that has seen everything and yet comes out with affirmation'.

Four noble truths of Buddhism are the truth of suffering, the truth of the cause of suffering, the truth of the end of suffering, and the truth of the path that leads to the end of suffering. More simply put, suffering exists, it has a cause, it has an end, and it has a cause to bring about its end. (). But the other tenets of Buddhism say, 'Everything is Temporary, Everything is Unpleasant, Everything is of its own Nature, Everything is Void.' That can be interpreted as, life is momentary, suffering is also momentary or transient and we need to use this present moment without wasting it for unnecessary activities.

(Reference:http://memyinnerthoughts.blogspot.com/2018/07/1182 -maha-vishnu-as-bauddha.html).

Another famous Buddhist quote from Thich Nhat Hanh that is relevant is: "Have compassion for all beings, rich and poor alike; each has their suffering. Some suffer too much, others too little."

Heinrich Zimmer says the following referring to Hinduism. He says that a spirit of unbounded optimism underlies all Indian philosophies. All Indian schools of thought say the solution to suffering is liberation, experiencing the 'Absolute', 'The Infinity', 'The Pure Consciousness'. Suffering transforms people and helps others and one's own welfare. My suffering led me to write this book and if it helps a few lives, my suffering would be worthwhile. I know that my suffering led me to recommend a few hundred screening colonoscopies and I know that it has resulted in early diagnosis of a few colon cancers. I hope it has prevented a few more colon cancers, making my suffering worthwhile. I confess that I realized the value of my suffering as I wrote this!

Karma theory to explain why bad things happen: Karma, in many ways, describes cause and effect relationships and it stands to logic. But what if one cannot trace a cause to an effect? The faiths that originated in India, such as Hinduism, Buddhism, Jainism, and Sikhism believe in Karma theory. These faiths also believe in the rebirth of the soul. The concept of rebirth helps continue the results of karma to the next birth.

In other words, certain events are attributed to the events in the previous births if no appropriate cause is found in this birth. The Bhagavad Gita on multiple occasions explains how offering the results of all activities to God helps attain everlasting peace without attachment to the fruits of action.

How is it to be understood that performing the same actions, some people are bound to material existence and others are released from material bondage? God answers that those who are unattached and unmotivated by material rewards are never bound by karma. But those craving rewards and obsessed with the desire to enjoy material pleasures become entangled in the reactions of work.

Persons who are "united in consciousness with God" relinquish the desire for the rewards of their actions, and instead engage in works for self-purification. Therefore, they soon attain divine consciousness and eternal beatitude. Those "desiring mundane rewards not beneficial to the soul" incited by cravings, lustfully desire the rewards of actions. The reactions of work performed in this consciousness bind such persons to the cycle of life and death.

These few sentences are from h, part of a beautiful commentary on the Gita by Swami Mukundananda. In chapter 5 (verse 13), God says that the embodied beings who are self-controlled and detached reside happily in the city of nine gates, free from thinking they are the doers or the cause of anything. God compares the body with its openings to a city of nine gates. The soul is like the king of the city, whose administration is carried out by the ministry of the ego, intellect, mind, senses, and life energy. The body consists of nine gates—two ears, one mouth, two nostrils, two eyes, anus, and genitals. In material consciousness, the soul residing with the body identifies itself with this city of nine gates. Within this body also sits the Supreme Lord, who is the controller of all living beings in the world.

When the soul establishes its connection with the Lord, it becomes free like Him, even while residing in the body.

In the preceding verse, Shree Krishna declared that the embodied soul is neither the doer nor the cause of anything. Then the question arises whether God is the actual cause of actions in the world? But the next verse states that neither the sense of doership nor the nature of actions comes from God, nor does He create the fruits of actions. All this is enacted by the modes of material nature. God controls the entire universe. Yet, He remains the non-doer. Had He been our director, there would not have been any bad events in this universe. Similarly, God is not responsible for our getting stuck with the sense of doership. If He had deliberately created the pride of doing in us, then again we could have blamed Him for our misdoings. He God did not cause cancer and also could not prevent it from coming.

Thus, renunciation of the sense of doership is the responsibility of the soul. All actions are performed by the body. But out of ignorance, the soul identifies with the body and becomes implicated as the doer of actions, which are in fact done by the physical body.

To summarize the answer to 'Why Me?', there is no good answer. There is a lot of randomness in this world and bad events randomly happen to people. It could happen to you too. The longer you live, the more likely it is going to happen to you. Unpleasant things happen even if you are a good person. Blaming yourself or anybody else or God or faith does not help. It is better to move on and ask, 'What can I do to make the situation better for me and my family?' Such challenges do indeed make us stronger. Even cancer patients indeed find ways to enjoy life and I encourage my patients to do so. The quote from Arthur Ashe, the tennis legend who developed AIDS, is very good. Ashe says, "If I were to say, 'God, why me?' about the bad things, then I should have said, 'God, why me?' about the good things that happened in my life." I have benefited from believing in God.

Some actions are meant to happen. The first verse of *Upadesha Sara* by Sri Ramana Maharshi explains that Karma is inert, meaning certain actions are inevitable, they are bound to happen. If we take certain consequences to be destined, it would be easy for us to accept a certain situation and then act in a way to get rid of it. This philosophy helps answer, 'Why Me?', it does not justify it. However hard we try not to ruminate on 'Why Me?', potential answers to this question can help us deal with cancer and also take measures to survive, prevent and liberate ourselves from cancer. Ruminating excessively on 'Why Me?' can be unhealthy and counterproductive. But rational thinking and scientific analysis on this certainly helps.

I have benefited from believing in non-dualism, which believes that there is God in me, right here, right now. It has given me access to experience God in this life rather than waiting to go to heaven after death to experience God. I have tried to convince myself that cancer and the terrible, excruciating pain that I suffered affected only my body and not me. This exercise of disowning cancer in my body and the pain was not entirely successful. I may not be that spiritually evolved to do that. The truth is when one is in pain, the only useful God is pain relief. For a hungry man, the only useful God is the one who brings food or food itself. For that reason, one of the saints (Swami Shivatmananda of Chinmaya Mission, Austin, and San Antonio), whom I know well, told me that 'non-dualism is a privilege.' However, it has been very empowering, gratifying, and joyful to experience God/Infinity in this life, every day, every moment of my life. It has been very enlightening to see God in everything and everybody. I pray that you get that experience of unveiling God in you. You have God in you, too!

iii. Prayer: Why? How? Transactional vs. non-transactional!

'Love, light, and education are the biggest multipliers; the more you share, the more it multiplies.'

- Anupkumar Shetty

"When I walk, I think I am circumambulating God; when I work, I think I am serving God; and when I sleep, I think I am offering him obeisance. In this manner, I perform no activity other than that which is offered to him."

-Kabir Das

I found integrating science, positive psychology and spirituality helpful. Traditionally, prayer is requesting God to do something good to help us. It could be 'curing of cancer', 'the next meal', 'some money', 'lots of money', 'love', 'lover', 'rain', 'better crops for a farmer', 'more business for a shopkeeper', 'life', or 'an organ that does not work in your body'. Patients sometimes pray to get a good doctor! I know many who are grateful to God for giving them compassionate and skilled doctors. I am grateful to God for sending the best doctors, nurses, and other healers to heal me and save my life. When you are practicing a dualistic religion, which includes most of the world religions including Christianity, Islam, Judaism, and a large number of Hindus and possibly Sikhs, Buddhists, and Jains, it is common to beg God for favors. However, a large number of Hindus are also non-dualists and 'qualified non-dualists.' The same thing is true of Sikhs, Buddhists, and Jains as well. I do not know enough about other religions like Bahá'í and other religions. There are some non-dualists in every religion. Many switch back and forth between non-dualism and dualism. Non-dualism can be very empowering in difficult situations because you are a small portion of God. In other words, non-dualists believe that 'Pure Consciousness is Brahman', 'the Self is Brahman', 'You are that' (you are that divine reality; 'That Thou Art'), and 'I am Brahman (God).' When God is in you or when you are God, there is no reason to worry. When you are God, whom do you pray? I pray to the God inside me! I pray that I realize the God in me! I pray to the God in me to take over my care! I completely surrender to the God in me and offer everything I do and eat to God. Historically the greatest scholars of non-dualism have been the greatest devotees of God. Hence devotion to God and the knowledge of non-dualism are not mutually exclusive. But a non-dualist prayer can be non-transactional, in that you don't have to beg for favors from God. All you beg is for God to be in you, manifest in you, run your life. You will automatically have a cancer-free and problem-free life. But, to be able to do this, you have to have the convincing knowledge that Brahman (God/Infinity) is in you. You have to have that conviction and confidence that the real 'I' is Brahman. To have that 'self-knowledge', one has to listen to divine teachings, one has to study it to ruminate on it, meditate upon it and internalize it. But if you don't have that divine self-knowledge with conviction, you can always fall back to love and devotion to God and worship God to help you and heal you. There is nothing wrong with it and that is what most people do.

Prayer should not be transactional if you are comfortable with it...

"Exploring the possibilities in life is trying to experience the God/Brahman/Infinity in this life."

This figure in the next page depicts the different ways and examples of prayers. Note that as we evolve spiritually, we stop begging God for favors and just desire to be closer to God till we realize that God is within us. It becomes easier once our basic needs are met. There is a parallel between the hierarchy of prayers that I have described here and the hierarchy of needs described by Abraham Maslow in his 1943 paper "A Theory of Human

Motivation" in the journal, Psychological Review. Maslow's hierarchy of needs include physiological needs followed by safety needs, belonging and love needs, esteem needs, cognitive needs, aesthetic needs, self-actualization and finally transcendence. Even positive psychology follows the hierarchy of needs!

Different Types and Levels of Prayers compared to Maslow's Hierarchy of Needs

HIERARCHY OF NEEDS	HIERARCHY OF PRAYERS
Physiological Needs	Requesting (praying) God for abundance in health, food, shelter, comfort, wealth, education, relationship (e.g. 'give me a pretty/handsome spouse, get my children married, give children, etc.) etc.
Safety Needs	Praying when in trouble: e.g. Please cure me from cancer, heart problem, diabetes, high blood pressure, etc., give me food, give me job, give me money, fix my relationship, give me good grades, give me admission to school of my choice, make the world healthy, get us through this pandemic, etc.
Belonging and Love Needs	
Esteem Needs	Praying God for blessing (less begging): e.g. 'Oh God, bless us'
Cognitive Needs	Praying God without praying for things: e.g. 'Oh God' (remembering God or chanting God's by various names or singing on God)
Aesthetic Needs	
Self Actualization	Realizing that God and I are inseparable (knowing that 'Consciousness is God', 'Self is God', 'You are God', 'I am God')
Transcendence	

Hierarchy of prayers and Maslow's heirarchy of needs

In one of the holy texts called *Srimad Bhagavatam*, one of the greatest devotees called Prahlada has described nine kinds of expressing the love of God (nine kinds of '*bhakti*'). They are 'listening' to the names and glories of God, 'chanting' the glories of God, 'remembering' God, 'serving' God, 'worshipping' God, 'offering obeisance' unto God, 'serving' as God's servant, developing 'friendship' with God and 'total surrender' to God. A given individual can express the love of God in more than one of these nine ways.

The Holy Bible describes seven prayers, viz, confession, salvation, release, submission, prayer, promise, and blessing.

I will repeat some concepts of prayer to reinforce them so you can meditate on them. The physical body in me tries to survive the risks of destruction from the different dangers in this world. The physical being in me wants to play a team sport by building the best team in the world to give me the best chance of conquering my cancer—best doctors, best nurses, best family, best friends, best hospital, etc. The physical person in me surrenders to the superpower in me to disown my body including cancer and my mind so I don't have to worry about it. The mental being in me acquires all the knowledge to do whatever it can be done to save my body from cancer. But the spiritual being in me itself is the omnipotent, omniscient Brahman/Infinity and hence I do not have to worry about cancer or any bodily problems.

The spiritual being in me realizes that it is only my physical body that gets sick and has the risk of dying; the spiritual being in me is never scared of getting sick, never scared of cancer, and never scared of death. The Brahman in me is aware that the real 'I' am the light of the lights, the strongest among the strong. The Brahman in me is aware that of the medicines I have the best medicine and of the Gods, I am the supreme and the only

God. I am time, I am timeless, and the beginning, middle and the end, and I'm fearless and all-loving and all-compassionate, I am self-effulgent, I am complete, I am the truth, I am 'THE ONE' and the only truth and the eternal truth, I am the 'Infinity'. When I know this I have nothing to worry about because what I see and what I feel is limited, temporary, and finite and hence not the infinite truth. The real truth is the pure consciousness in me. Hence when I pray all I have to do is to surrender to the God in me, offer my body and mind to God, and lose the boundary between myself and God and experience the God in me. In chapter 2 of the Bhagavad Gita, Shree Krishna says that the real me cannot be cut, cannot be made wet, cannot be burned, it is eternal, it is all-pervading. We should do our duties not so much with passion, but with tranquility (equanimity of mind) as a service to God. If we do everything including eating, breathing, drinking, taking medicines as service to God, we would only do the right thing, we would only do the best thing in the world.

To be able to trust in what scriptures and teachers tell us is, in itself, a wonderful blessing. Because only this trust will make it possible for us to be able to understand who we in fact are. That which is one, free, all-pervasive, and eternal. Trust is very important for those who pray. Trust is love and devotion. In fact, devotion to God is not that difficult because all you need is trust and love towards God. Shree Krishna says in the Gita (4:39) that those whose faith is deep and who have practiced controlling their mind and senses attain divine knowledge. Through such transcendental knowledge, they quickly attain everlasting supreme peace, the peace that God will take care of everything.

I am deliberately mixing up non-dualism and dualism because they don't have to be mutually exclusive. Earlier, I said that trust is paramount in dualistic prayer. But even in non-dualism, you have to utterly, totally, absolutely relinquish the one who you take yourself to be, striving to feel your light of lights within you. To let the body go, you need trust. The one and only reliable one to place your trust in is the divine. Everything and everyone will fail at some point. But, please pray if you wish. It does not matter how. There are no rules of prayer. Pray in a way that empowers you. Sometimes surrendering to the Supreme God/Brahman and allowing yourself to be small empowers you. Sometimes, knowing that you are inside God empowers you. Sometimes, knowing that you are God, that you are magnanimous, will empower you. Be small, be big, or be magnanimous depending upon the situation, as God Hanuman did. In Ramayana, a Hindu epic, God Hanuman became small like a mosquito and big like a giant, depending upon the situation. He lived as a servant of God, a part of God, or simply as God himself, depending upon the situation.

You can be thankful for every little thing and every big thing you have and you don't have. You can be thankful to your family and friends you have; you can be thankful to your healthcare providers. You can count every blessing. When you practice gratitude, you will learn to be happy with what you have and not be unhappy with your problems. You will always find reasons to be happy when you start counting your blessings. When you learn to practice gratitude to the Consciousness, Brahman, God, Infinity, you will learn to love God. You will not be angry at God despite having problems.

You will find peace within yourself. You will find that infinite consciousness within you. You will find spiritual healing. You will find God right within you, right now, right in this life. God ceases to be an after-death dream. It becomes an experience in this life. Swami Dayananda says: "Prayer is invoking grace as well as an act that is a simple autosuggestion." Prayer does help. Try yourself in whichever way suits your beliefs.

Chapter Six

After Cancer (Contd..): Dealing With Fecal Incontinence, Reason to Live, Staring at Death

iv. Living with incontinence

I am incontinent. I have fecal incontinence. I have been incontinent ever since I had the 'big surgery'. It became obvious the day I had my 'ileostomy' reversed and the need for the fecal pouch removed. I can control urination. I thank God for that! It sounds difficult to live with incontinence. It is difficult. More than difficult, even though it comes with challenges, it is a nuisance, it is inconvenient. It is humbling, it makes you feel powerless.

These are some highlights of how I live with fecal incontinence:

1. I wear diapers: If I get a bowel movement during the day or night and if the diaper gets dirty it has to be changed as soon as possible. Don't think that one can leave the dirty diaper for hours just because they are diapers. Don't think that one can sleep through the night with dirty diapers. No, you can't. It only protects what you wear over the diaper and what you sleep on. It does not prevent the person from being uncomfortable. It helps the clothes from getting wet if you urinate or have a bowel movement. Do you know why babies cry and the elderly scream when the diaper is wet? That is because it is very uncomfortable having a soiled diaper. Many people don't know that. Caregivers need to know this. Nurses and patient care technicians in hospitals and nursing homes need to know this. I have heard caregivers say with a sigh, 'Thank God for the diapers'! Yes, we have to be thankful for the diapers. Because they protect the clothes, the bedsheets, the mattresses, and the beds. It does reduce the caregiver burden. Diapers give some time before you attend to the incontinent person. It gives you minutes, not hours without keeping the person uncomfortable. If you wait long enough, even the clothes and bedsheets get soiled. Sometimes people develop diaper rash and bed sores! So, beware! I am fortunate that I can take care of myself when my diaper is messy. Thankfully it does not happen often. It happens more often when my diet changes while traveling. I tend to eat a lot more when I am traveling and end up paying a price too. One of my doctors told me to eat just once a day so I will have fewer stools. No, I can't do that. To avoid the need to change diapers frequently, I put toilet paper inside my diapers. If I have an involuntary bowel movement, all I have to change is the toilet paper and not the diaper after I clean myself in most situations unless the situation is very messy! This approach is both environmentally friendly, cost-effective, and convenient.

Fecal incontinence can give you a diaper rash that can be painful. I have found applying coconut oil very helpful. It is very soothing and possibly helps healing. You can try any product that works for you. Your doctor may be able to recommend you one. Most doctors may not know what to recommend. I have had to consult a wound care specialist, Dr Applewhite, once when I was desperate. Wound care specialists are very good at taking care of 'skin interruptions and wounds'. Lidocaine jelly applied topically on the rash does not help. It hurts a lot, it burns! I usually carry extra diapers in my backpack all the time. If I am traveling outside the US I prefer to carry a roll or two of soft toilet paper. During one of my pilgrimage trips in Sri Sailam, India, I ran out of toilet paper. My friend, Prasad's wife Janaki rescued me by getting it from a random hotel. God came in my life as Janaki that particular day to help me. If I am flying anywhere I usually carry the enema bag and travel size petroleum jelly in the carry-on baggage. The disposable enema bags are hard to find in stores because there are not many people with fecal incontinence who give themselves enemas. There are times I have given myself enema inside the plane. That is very traumatic mentally because I have to stay inside the restroom for an hour fearing that somebody will knock on the door! It is not fair to other travelers and be sure that somebody will knock at your door. It has happened to me!

2. Enema or colon irrigation: I give myself an enema every day, at least six days a week if my weekend is free. Be careful in choosing the enema bags. The red rubber enema bags that many hospitals use have a rough tip that is difficult for daily use. Moreover, the bag is opaque and you cannot see how much water has gone in, you cannot even see if the water is flowing in. If I cannot see the water level, I lose control over what I am doing! Controlling the controllable is very important to most human beings, more so for people who have lost control over things that they had before. For those reasons, I don't use the red rubber reusable enema bags. I use clear plastic non-reusable bags. The tip that goes inside the anus is smooth and you can monitor the flow of water since the bag is see-through plastic! The tip has to be lubricated with some lubricant such as petroleum jelly. Vaseline® is a standard brand, but many stores have their own brands and it is available at the baby toiletry supplies section in the stores. I worry about using petroleum jelly every day that touches my skin around the anus. Petroleum is considered carcinogenic, but I don't know if petroleum jelly is carcinogenic. I am looking for a non-petroleum-based lubricant. But

I have not looked hard enough! The enema bags are only available in very few places. I buy mine from Dougherty's medical supply store in North Dallas and from Amazon.com. The only store that sells these enema bags in Dallas ran out of them once and I nearly panicked. I went to several stores in Dallas and I could not find them. I also called my sister in Houston immediately to look for them. My life is very dependent on the enema bags and it would be very different and difficult for me without them. I have the red rubber enema bags as a backup. Fortunately, I found the plastic disposable enema bags online at Amazon.com and I bought enough supplies to last a few years. Even though they are supposed to be disposable, I can reuse them several times so I can be environmentally friendly by reducing plastic usage and being cost-conscious.

My insurance company does not cover the expenses of diapers and enema bags. But some insurances, especially Medicare, may cover it. Please check with your insurance company if they will pay for them.

Ever since I started doing colon irrigation/enema, my life has been great. I don't get frequent 'accidents' (involuntary bowel movements) and I don't have the pain in the belly that I experienced for several years. I was generally using six to seven diapers a week. Of late I have become more confident of not wearing diapers on certain days if it feels good, but I always carry diapers and a pair of pants in my backpack as a backup.

3. Dietary changes for better bowel management and cancer prevention: I have had to make some dietary changes to avoid frequent bowel movements and prevent cancer. According to Tricia Petzold of the University of Utah, cancer prevention happens in the kitchen. Lentil soup (also called 'dal' in Hindi) is a very integral part of Indian food. I have had to avoid this to a large extent except in very limited amounts if I have time and access to restrooms. I avoid chickpeas as well in all forms. I still eat some 'rajma' (kidney beans) and some 'dal' here and there. My wife cooks them so well that it is hard to resist. You will learn the cancer diet and foods to avoid from trial and error after a few messy situations.

I have a very simple cancer diet and incontinence diet. Here is my cancer diet cookbook for you:

Breakfast: My usual breakfast is smoothie and tea. If I am bored of smoothies, I have a liberal amount of peanut butter or almond butter with bread, apple, or banana.

Smoothie with two fruits (e.g.: one apple and one banana, it is alright to put strawberries, blueberries, any berries, mangoes, papaya, pineapple, raisins, almost any seasonal fruit), two servings of organic green leafy vegetables of my choice (kale/tender spinach/cucumber/celery/etc.), a handful of almonds (about 10-15) or 10-15 cashews (sometimes I eat pistachios or walnuts as well), a scoop or more of protein powder (I use Orgain® organic plant-based powder), about 500-700 ml of water to bring the level to ~90% of the level of all contents in the blending jar; blend all these together and drink it fresh. You can use coconut water instead of water if you want to spend more money. Don't use milk, sugar, sweetener, or syrup.

Optional additions are small pieces of ginger (1/4 inch or less), 1/4 teaspoonful of turmeric powder, or small pieces of turmeric root, parsley, thyme, basil, or cilantro (coriander leaves). A few drops of honey are okay. Please don't add spoonfuls of honey. When it comes to green leafy vegetables, one handful or one tennis ball-sized serving is considered one serving.

I usually add one or two teaspoons of flax seeds, flax seed powder, and/or chia seeds. Rarely, I add one or two dates if I am not adding honey or raisins.

I avoid peas and chickpeas. You can add peanut butter or almond butter as the source of protein and fat instead of protein powder.

I have tried different juicers and blenders. I find Nutribullet® and Vita-mix® most user-friendly and I mostly use Nutribullet®. They are easier to use and easier to clean.

In addition, I make about 500 ml (~16 ounces) of hot tea with 50% water, 50% milk (2%), two teaspoons of black tea powder, or two-three teabags (black tea, Lipton®, Earl gray®, or English breakfast; don't put herbal tea/lemon tea/peppermint tea since they curdle the milk). It is alright to add ginger or cardamom to tea. You can add a small amount (less than one spoonful) of sugar if your health permits.

When I am traveling I avoid anything with lentils. I can have anything with cereals (rice, corn, wheat), quinoa, sesame seeds, peanuts, almonds, cashews, pecans, cornmeal, cornbread, or flaxseed meal. I can also have anything with eggs, tomatoes, potatoes, and onion. That means I can have omelets, scrambled eggs, boiled eggs, or 'sunny side up' and potatoes. There is some link between colon cancer and high egg consumption. For that reason, I limit my intake of eggs. I probably eat about four eggs in a month. This is what I usually have if I am in a hotel.

I can have any of the fruits, bread, and juices. But remember that white bread is not as healthy as whole grain bread. Juice is not healthy, fruit is better. Too much fruit gives you more sugar and that is not good if you are a diabetic or overweight. High-fiber fruits such as apples, berries, and grapefruits are healthier than low-fiber fruits such as melons, bananas, pineapples, oranges, and mangoes. Remember that grapefruits interact with statin drugs that reduce cholesterol.

Meals: I usually have rice, chapati, and vegetables. I have a liberal amount of vegetables. For proteins, I have cottage cheese (paneer), nuts, fish or eggs, and some beans. I don't eat any meat other than fish, seafood, and eggs, three to four days a month. If you like you can have some meat in moderation. Generally, animal-based proteins are considered not healthy for anybody, especially for the colon and the brain, and the mind. If I was able to tolerate lentils, I would have totally avoided fish and eggs as well.

If I am eating Mediterranean food, I eat salad, pita bread, and fish. I try to avoid hummus and falafel because it is made of chickpeas even though I like them a lot and I am drooling now! But I don't get to eat Mediterranean food that often anyways. I am from India and Indian food is entirely different from Middle Eastern food. For the geographically challenged readers, India is not in the Middle East!

I don't restrict milk, yogurt, and cheese. The only cheese I like is paneer. I only eat plain yogurt with rice. Sweetened yogurt is not on my menu.

Drinks: I limit my drinks to smoothies and tea in the morning, and water for the rest of the day. I largely avoid juice to reduce my sugar intake. I entirely avoid sodas, all the carbonated and non-carbonated sugary drinks. I think that nobody should drink any sugary, carbonated, or non-carbonated drinks. I feel that they caused the epidemic of diabetes and obesity that we are seeing all over the world, especially in India and China. I feel that sugary drinks have hurt more people than anything else in the world.

So, my standard recommendation (not prescription!) to everybody is *no sodas, no juice, no sugar, no sweets, limit on salt and avoid beef and pork. Let two-thirds of your plate have vegetables every meal every day.* That means no desserts, no ice creams, no cakes, no candies! You can follow this 100% or close to that! It will serve you well in life. This is good for everybody, not just for cancer prevention.

4. Travel: I request for an aisle seat while flying to be able to use the toilet if I have to without inconveniencing others. If I am flying to India or back from India to the US, I make sure I give myself an enema a few hours before the travel begins because travel time is usually about 24 hours. There are times I have given myself an enema in the restrooms in the airport. This is a little bit unpleasant because restrooms in the airport usually have water faucets in the common area and you have to fill the enema bags with water in the common area. If you are sensitive to what people will think if they see you fill the enema bags, you will either have to get tough or not do it. One thing you want to avoid is having frequent bowel movements in the diaper and not having access to the toilet. You really don't risk having bowel movements while flying. On a few occasions, desperate occasions, I have given myself an enema in the toilets on the plane. It is not recommended. You should always carry the enema bag and lubricant in your carry-on luggage in case you get stranded in a place without your check-in luggage. Once I was in a hotel in Bahrain after I missed my connecting flight because my initial flight got delayed. I had no access to my checked-in bags for another 40 hours. Thankfully I had an enema bag with me to keep me continent! Readymade enemas that you get in pharmacies don't serve my purpose. They are meant for constipation, not for colon irrigation.

5. Planning the day: It takes about 90 minutes to give myself an enema, clean up and take shower. This is not something you can do in a hurry. For that reason, it takes longer for me to get ready for work in the mornings. I had to make some changes at work. I had to choose to work more in the office and less in the hospital since the office opens at 9:00 a.m. My colleagues at Dallas Nephrology Associates were kind enough to accommodate my needs. I compensated for the favor by choosing to work late in the evenings so I can stay productive. If mornings are unpredictable such as on the days after working at night, I give myself an enema at night.

6. Don't let incontinence stop you: Incontinence never stopped me. I did many things that I had never done before. I walked uphill to Tirupati temple, Sabarimalai Ayyappa temple, Vaishno Devi temple, Kunjara Giri temple, and many places considered sacred for Hindus, which involved walking variable distances up the hills meditating and transcending to divinity. My Shabarimalai trip had several interruptions due to my incontinence. Part of this trip was barefoot hiking, which went fine. This is a very humbling visit because everybody has to manage with minimal amenities with no warm water to shower and no beds to sleep on. You have to take a cold bath and sleep on a concrete floor with a bedsheet. Eight of us slept in one room and shared a bathroom. Of course, there is no air conditioning. I circumambulated the mountains of Tiruvannamalai in southern India meditating on God in the form of Arunachala Shiva. This was my equivalent of hiking to Mount Kailash in the Himalayas since I may not be able to go there due to incontinence. I worshipped and meditated at the Ashram of Bhagavan Ramana Maharshi, a sage of the 20th century who propagated non-dualistic philosophy whom I revere a lot. I worshipped at the Arunachala temple where Lord Shiva manifests as fire, one of the five primary elements. It is so real here that the praying area near the shrine is so hot. 'fire' element tooThis temple is magnanimous and magnificent. I am not sure how anybody could have built this without cranes and modern technology that we have access to today. It could be either divine blessings or technologies that existed in ancient India. Many of these temples can easily be the wonders of the world. I also visited the Taj Mahal. I visited Mathura, the birthplace of God Krishna when he manifested as a human being. Part of this structure was invaded and destroyed by the Muslim kings and a mosque has been built there. It is interesting to see a Hindu Temple and a mosque on two sides of one building! My drive to Mathura was also interrupted several times due to incontinence. I took a dip and prayed at the holy Golden Temple, Amritsar, India, the holiest of the places for the Sikhs. I also visited the Vatican, Saint Mary's Church in Mahim, Mumbai, and Haji Ali Darga in Mumbai with reverence. I also tried surfing the oceans in Hawaii and Puerto Rico, rope riding in Puerto Rico, snorkeling in the caverns of Mexico, and hiking in and around

Machu Picchu, Peru. I prayed and recited a set of verses on 'Sun God' (*Aditya Hrdayam*) at the Sun Temple in Machu Picchu.

There can be no life without the Sun. If there is no Sun, there would be no day and there would be no night. There would be only darkness. If there is no sunlight, there would be no living beings on the earth. Imagine living with 'Sun in your eyes.' You would see everything that the Sun has access to. You would never see darkness. Yes, you are reading this right! Sun never sees darkness or a shadow. Sun only sees light. Sun never sees darkness. That is how important the Sun is. If you see divinity in everything and everybody, you certainly would see divinity in the Sun. This is why many worship the Sun. Many Hindus worship the Sun. Aztecs worshipped Sun God. Incans worshipped Sun God. I have visited the Mayan temples in Progresso, Tulum, and Chichen Itza in Mexico. I also went to the highest place in Europe, Titlis, and rolled around in the snow like a baby partly to relieve my pain in the belly and partly to celebrate it since this trip had to be cancelled a week before the trip due to small bowel obstruction and rebooked after two or three days when I got better!

v. Strong reason for living

I went through a lot of pain during chemotherapy and after surgery. One of the side effects of chemotherapy with 5-FU (5 fluorouracil) is frequent loose bowel movements. And one of the side effects of radiation is that it makes the tissues swollen and fragile. Colon has no pain sensation, but my cancer was very close to the anus, which has nerve fibers carrying pain sensation. Radiation causes damage to the tissues around cancer and causes frequent bowel movements. Having bowel movements those days was literally like pulling a jute rope over a raw wound. After so many years, I can still feel it! Later on, I had more pain after surgery. That pain was so bad that I could not sit upright for almost six weeks after surgery. For that reason, I could not drive a car. It is not a good idea to take narcotic pain medicines and drive with pain. You cannot concentrate. I have done a little bit of such driving and caught myself driving through a red light a few times. I do not recommend anyone driving with pain especially if you are taking narcotics for pain relief. I have experienced more pain since then, especially in the first five years after surgery till I started treating myself with an enema every day.

About one year after the diagnosis, I was asking myself if it was worth going through the pain of chemotherapy, radiation, and surgery. I felt that it was not worth it unless one has a good reason to live. I had a good reason to live. I had to financially support my wife and young children at least till they get some education to be independent. I think parents provide emotional support to children as well. I owed my wife and children that support. Of course, my other family members including my parents, siblings, in-laws, and others including my friends would have liked me to live. I know of some elderly people in their eighties who like to live to financially support their children and grandchildren. Some people like to live till their grandchildren graduate or get married or have children. We all have different reasons to live. Many are just scared of dying and want to live because they don't want to die. They express gratitude every day because they're 'standing above the dirt'. In my faith, death is like discarding a shirt. In Hinduism, the soul (*Atma*) or the real 'I' never dies. Only the physical body dies. Once the body dies, the soul occupies another body or merges with God. This teaching gave me a lot of comfort. For that reason, I was not really scared of dying, but at the same time, I did not want to die so I could support my wife and children. I realized that dying was easy for the person who dies. Because once you die, you are no more in pain and no more in suffering. It is the family who suffers. Sometimes we don't realize who we are crying for when a loved one dies. We should be crying for the remaining family members rather than the ones who pass on. But it is hard for most of us, including myself.

"All you have to do is get better. That is your only choice." Sudha M.

Desire to win the battle of cancer is extremely important if you want to survive. At the age of 41 years, being the sole breadwinner for the family, I did not have a choice of not winning. I had to live to support my young family in all different ways. I had a 35 years-old wife and two young kids aged 10 and 5. My mother-in-law reminded me the first day that I had young children who needed me. My good friend, Sudha called me and gave me this very profound advice. It might sound logical and easy, but to me, it was very profound. She said, 'Anup, all you have to do is get better. That is your only choice'. She did not say, 'Anup, I am sorry that you got cancer, but don't worry, you will get better'. Isn't this what most people tell you if you are sick? That is not what Sudha said. She said, 'Anup, you have to get better. That is your only choice'. This reminds me of the 'Limca' ad in Hindi in the 80s and 90s in India: *'Yahee hai right choice, baby!'* (This is the right choice, baby!). My only choice was to get better. Another good friend of mine, Shannon told me the week before the surgery. 'You better do well after the surgery! We have had enough bad news during the last few months.' Two of my best friends and colleagues had passed on in a plane crash 10 days before my surgery and another colleague was very sick (he is doing well since then) after a ruptured appendix around that time. My point is Sudha and Shannon empowered me to get better and I felt strong. Even though they said what they said, this is what I heard from them. **'Arise, awake, stop not till your goal is reached'** (as Swami Vivekananda said). This is what I heard from God Krishna, 'Arise Anup, get off from faintheartedness, this does not befit you, go and fight the just war'. (Bhagavad Gita Ch 2:3). There are few examples of integrating positive psychology in my life.

My closest friend and spiritual advisor, Raju has had an important role in my life. He introduced me to a hymn called *Hanuman Chalisa* that many Hindus know. *Hanuman Chalisa* is a hymn consisting of 40 verses about God Hanuman. Hanuman is an incarnation of God Shiva and is the epitome of physical strength, humility, knowledge, public speaking, servitude, leadership, healing, and divine power. Lord Hanuman is believed to have told the God who came to this earth as King Rama, 'at the body level I am your servant, at the level of 'life energy' I am a part of you and at the Divine level, I and you are the same'. This concept worked very well to empower me. I have seen myself in all these three roles at different times of my life, depending upon the need, my mental state, and the ability to withdraw from the mundane world. I am thankful to Raju for teaching me this concept. Moreover, I felt that it was my duty and responsibility to my young family to get better. My children Krishna and Eesha and my wife, Mala were the biggest agents of empowerment for me. That empowerment and the sense of responsibility led to the desire to win this game. I very well know that winning or losing was not in my hands. But working towards a win was in my hands.

Like the holy Gita, *Song of God,* says, 'You claim ownership to your duties, not to the fruits of action and one should not give company to inaction' (2:47). The latter part of this teaching, 'one should not give company to inaction' is extremely important. So one should act efficiently with all the skills one has with equanimity of mind to give the best chance to win. The keywords in this sentence are 'act', 'all the skills', 'efficient', 'equanimity', 'win', and 'do not give company to inaction'. Act, you must. Everybody is helplessly driven to act. One should not give company to inaction. I know of people who don't take treatment for fear of side effects of treatment and say that 'Lord will heal me'. We know that not everyone with cancer or any serious problem gets better. We have to do our part to 'help' the Lord to heal us, for the Lord to transform us from weakness to strength, weight to light, illness to wellness, and from cancer to no cancer. This transformative statement is inspired from the prayer, 'Lead me from Untruth to Truth, Ignorance to Knowledge and Mortality to Immortality' ['*Asatoma* (*asat*=untruth) *Satgamaya* (*sat*=truth), *tamasoma* (*tamas* =inertia=darkness=ignorance) *jyotirgamaya* (*jyoti* = light =knowledge), *mrtyorma* (*mrt* = death) *amrtamgamaya* (*amrt* = immortality = elixir of immortality)'], a famous prayer from Rig Veda, a Hindu scripture that I recite and meditate upon every day of my life. President Obama used to frequently quote this prayer, whenever he used to address Hindu festivals. Everything we do daily is about this transformation from bad to good in life. It is about transforming carbon into diamond! Remember that diamond is carbon too, so is charcoal. Diamonds are so clear, hard, shining, and sparkling. It is all in you. That infinite strength is in you. Infinity is in you. God is in you! In fact, 'You Are That'. It is about the journey from adversity to a new normalcy. The new normalcy is often different from the original normalcy. These are few examples of applying spirituality for my recovery.

"Your willingness to live is a major factor for your survival. A strong reason to live makes the efforts even stronger and helps you to survive in the toughest situations."

vi. Staring at death and staring at immortality

When I had cancer, I did not know if I was going to survive. People around me did not know either. But, generally, the first word that comes to people's minds when they hear 'cancer' is 'death'. Many had written me off.

People were concerned about who would take care of my children when they heard that I had cancer. That did not empower me! But those who had this fear were very loving human beings, they just did not know what to say. A friend told my wife that she would pray for miracles. When I heard this, what I heard was 'only a miracle can save me, otherwise I am destined to die'. Our mind is strange. The same words mean different things for different people. Sometimes the intonation changes the meaning of the same sentence. Brian Tracy gives the example of how saying 'I love you' could mean different things depending upon how you say it and whom you say that. It could mean 'I love you' or 'I don't love you' depending upon how it is told. It could mean 'I only love you and nobody else', 'Do you really mean I love you?', 'Why would I love you?' and many other things. My friend, Professor Gautam Suresh, a specialist in treating newborns and a public speaker, once explained to us about different ways of saying, 'I didn't do that' in different intonations and conveying different things. Try it out! It could mean different things like, 'I really did not do that', 'I did not do *that*, but I did something else', '*I* did not do that, but someone else did that', 'do you really mean that I did that?', 'why would I do that?' and few other things depending upon which word you stress and where you paused.

Preparing to die is something we all have to do before we get sick. The only preparation that I had done was that I had a reasonable life insurance policy and I had a living will. It is recommended to have a power of attorney to designate people to make healthcare decisions if we are unable to make those decisions. More importantly, one should talk to the family members when one can and explain to them your choices because immediate family members can overrule the advanced directives.

How did I prepare for death? Actually, I did not. But I did do a few things. I invited my insurance agent to my home and had him explain to my wife what the procedure is if I were to die. Thanks to Jim Stevens from Northwest Mutual for being very gracious and humane in coming to my home. He explained to my wife and me the different ways to draw money in the event of my death. I showed my wife where the life insurance policy is. I also told her the passwords for my bank accounts and retirement accounts, which have changed since then! I explained to her my wishes. I showed her my living will. Some people make their funeral arrangements. I did not. 'Death planning' is done more in the western world than in India. I may have thought that I was not that likely to die of cancer at that time! I was not planning to die that easily! I was not planning to die young!

On a lighter note, I did think of death. I was thinking of how my funeral would be if I were to die. I have seen funerals in India where usually 150 – 500 people attend. I was thinking that my funeral would be so boring in Dallas with only a handful of people. I thought that it would be a sad thing for me to die so far away from family members! I thought that my good friend Mahesh Shetty, a very eloquent speaker, would do the eulogy! I also realized that death is easy for the person who dies and harder for the family members who are left behind.

Looking back, it is crazy and creepy! How does it matter how many people attend my funeral after I am dead and gone? But it looks like I had the wish that most of my close family relatives should attend my funeral and remember me as a good human being. In a way I still do! I am extremely blessed with very loving family members both from my side and my wife's side. I have few who do special prayers or start fasting if I get extra bowel movements. That is how much they love me! I am extremely blessed with very good friends who actually are the 'first responders' if something catastrophic were to happen to me. Sometimes I wonder if I deserve it. Nevertheless, it is a nice feeling to be poured with love that I have the privilege of.

Every adult should have a living will and medical power of attorney. This has to be done when we are in good health. Once you have the living will and medical power of attorney, you have to discuss it with your close family members including those without power of attorney. The ones who have the power of attorney should have a copy of these legal documents.

The more and more I thought of the logistics of death, the more I thought of families which have lost their loved ones. It was an amazing revelation for me. Death is one of the most certain things for the one who is born. Everybody who is born will definitely die someday. I realized that death is easy for the person who dies. We don't know what happens to us after we die. If I die, I am dead and gone! I have few options about how to die gracefully. I have the option of explaining to my nearest family members if I want to be kept on resuscitative measures. I have the option of choosing to be in hospice to have a dignified death with less suffering. I have the option of dying at the hospital, nursing home, or home. I have the option to plan my funeral before death. I can communicate with my family if I want to be cremated or buried. I have the option of where to have the funeral. Not every breath one takes is worth the suffering that comes with it. Most die before their heart stops beating. In other words, life ends a few days to weeks before we die in most situations. I think it is better to die a few days or weeks or even months earlier to avoid the pain and suffering that comes at the end of life. It will be better for the family and society too. More one suffers at the end of life, the harder it is for the person and harder it is for the family members. Healthcare in the intensive care units in the hospitals is very painful and expensive too. It will reduce the health care costs that we are struggling to contain if we spend our last few days of life at home with our family rather than spending those days in the intensive care units with tubes going through all the holes we have, breathing tube, feeding tube, rectal tube, urinary catheter, catheters in the veins and arteries!

It would have been nice if we could cut the suffering during the last few weeks of our lives! But the problem is that none of us know our expiration dates! This topic is outside the scope of this book. But changing terminal care to compassionate care is a good option to allow the person to die with dignity.

"My body is mortal, but the real 'I', my soul is immortal"

"Ye, Children of Immortal Bliss," said Swami Vivekananda.

I would like to discuss rebirth since we are studying death. Some faiths believe in rebirth and some don't. Many people believe in rebirth even if their religion does not. I am not an expert on all faiths. But I have been studying the Hindu religion that I follow and have authored the book, *Hinduism Simplified.* Hindus believe in rebirth. We believe in the immortal nature of the soul, the Atman. We believe that the physical body is mortal and it gets changed like a garment on the soul that is immortal. Your soul is the real 'you' and your body is not the real 'you'. When we 'die', only the body dies, but our soul doesn't. That is why I said we are 'kind of' reborn. In reality, it is not really a rebirth. The soul moves on from one body to another or is 'reborn' in another body. When the real 'I' is not going to die, why am I worried about death? This is a very powerful concept that gives a lot of courage to face the death of our mortal body. This is the power of the concept of 'non-duality', where the soul is considered a part of God. A good example given is the wave and the ocean. The ocean is like God and the wave is like the soul. Both the wave and the ocean are made of water and they are one and the same; water is the Universal God in this example.

Advanced care planning: Death planning is not the same as planning to die!

When you have a big surgery, there is a finite chance of bad outcomes including death. Indians usually do not do funeral arrangements before death. It is not in our culture! In the US, when you are admitted, don't be surprised if someone asks you if you have done your funeral arrangements. It is in the list of questions they are supposed to ask before surgery. They will also ask if you would like to be resuscitated if your heart were to stop. Generally, surgeons and anesthesiologists would like to revive you if the heart were to stop during or immediately after the surgery. In fact, I found out that veterinary surgeons ask the same question if your pet is going to need surgery. I found out recently when my dog, Sophie, needed an emergency surgery. My point is that you should not get offended if you are asked such questions.

Death, sometimes, is the end of pain and suffering. There is no suffering after death. Nobody knows what happens after death. It is the family that suffers after the untimely death of a family member. I had a decent life insurance policy and I thought that my family would be comfortable from a financial standpoint of leading an average life if I were to die. Thinking of all these things, I thought that it would be alright if I were to die. But I wanted to live to support my young family. Most faiths of the world including Christians, Muslims, Jews, and many Hindus believe that we go to heaven or hell after death. Hindus believe in rebirth if one has not accumulated enough good things/karma to permanently merge with God. Some Hindus (followers of Yoga or Sankhya philosophy), Buddhists, and Jains believe that one experiences God or Nothingness (also called *shoonya* or *NirvaaNa* by the Buddhists) in this life. Some rare people admit having such a mystic experience where they talk to God. But a lot of Hindus believe that they are part of the big Universal God like a wave in the big ocean and that God is available to be experienced in everyday life in oneself and everybody and everything! Non-dualists believe that the real 'I', pure consciousness, never dies, it is fearless, birthless, deathless, all loving, all compassionate, self-effulgent, all-pervading, eternal, ultimate, ONE truth that witnesses the 'self' manifest in the body and mind in the wake, sleep, and dream states. They believe that the real consciousness is God. 'I am He', 'I am That', 'I am Brahman', 'You are that divine reality' are some of the expressions to describe this relationship with God! Most Hindus go back and forth between being dualists and non-dualists. I should not fear death! And to a large extent, I did not think of death even though I made my life insurance agent explain the 'death benefits' to my wife! Life insurance agents have a strange way of calling the amount of money life is insured as the 'death benefit'. It is so creepy to express that a person gets 'benefited' from the death of a family member! But that is the transactional world for us! Even death is a transaction!

The secret of death: Nachiketha story

There is a story in one of the sacred Hindu texts called '*Kathopanishad*'. The highlight of the text is the dialogue between a boy called Nachiketha and the God of Death. Apparently, the boy was sent to the God of death as a punishment by his angry father. Pleased by the little boy for waiting for him at the gate of the God of Death without food and water for three days, the God of Death asks the boy to ask for three boons. The third boon that the boy asks is the 'secret of death'. When the God of Death resists answering this question by offering him abundant wealth and kingdom, pretty women, long life, and all the pleasures of earth and heaven, the boy insists on an answer to his question of the secret of death. He tells the 'God of Death', 'keep all those pleasures to yourself and answer my question' and that 'as long as there is you, the God of Death, there is no meaning to all the pleasures and wealth'. The God of Death is very pleased with the wisdom of the boy who knew that worldly pleasures are transitory and explains to him about the eternal truth of the 'Self/Atman/Soul/Infinity' and transitory nature of the body and mind. The God of Death defines the innermost essence of our being. It is extremely subtle and hence cannot be heard or felt or smelled or tasted like any ordinary object. It never dies. It has no beginning or end. It is unchangeable. Realizing this Supreme Reality, man escapes from death and attains everlasting life. Thus the God of Death, the teacher, has gradually led Nachiketa to a point where he can reveal to him the secret of death. The boy had thought that there was a place where he could stay and become immortal. But the God of Death shows him that immortality is a state of consciousness and is not gained so long as man clings to name and form, or perishable objects. What dies? Form. Therefore the formful man dies; but not that which dwells within. He goes on to tell that those who do not know this truth go from 'death to death' and those who know this truth appreciate the immortal nature of the real self, also called 'Atman', and do not fear death. Knowing the nature of the 'Self' takes away the fear of death. Knowing that 'I' am 'Infinity', why fear death? Knowing that 'you' are 'Infinity', why fear death? That is the power of Infinity! Knowing this truth gives us the courage to stare at 'death' and live a fearless life. As pure water poured into more pure water becomes 'one', so also is it with the Self of an illumined knower who becomes one with the Supreme.

It is from this Upanishad text that Swami Vivekananda addressed people, 'Ye, children of Immortal bliss!' Knowing that we are beings of immortal bliss helps us stare at 'death' without fear of death. Incidentally, it is also from this text that he came up with his famous quote, 'Rise, Awake, Stop not till your goal is reached.' This is another example of how I integrated spirituality and positive psychology in navigating cancer with the power of Infinity.

SECTION 3: PREVENTION OF CANCER

Chapter Seven

Genesis of Cancer

i. The mathematical way of genesis, treatment, and prevention of cancer

*E*verything matters in life, be it a healthy diet, exercise, *adequate sleep, adequate rest, regular meditation, regular prayers, commitment to being happy, and an attitude of gratitude!*

If you are mathematically challenged, you can skip this chapter. If you like mathematics like I do, you are welcome to read this chapter and I hope it makes sense. I have had mixed reviews from my reviewers about this chapter before publishing the book. I don't know why I developed cancer. My dear 'uncle' Mr. Krishnamurthy Malladi told me not to ask 'Why me?' I did not ask 'Why me?' and cry over it. But we all have a curious scientist within us; there is one in me too. I think I have an explanation as to why I got cancer and why people get cancer. Incidentally, one saint asked me if I went through a prolonged phase of difficulty in life. I did have a period of extreme physical and mental stress for two years in my late 20s. That just confirmed what I was thinking. Let us figure out why one gets cancer even if you are not a scientist, doctor, or mathematician. Let us do it mathematically since it stands for logic. All you need to understand is simple additions, subtractions, multiplication, and division that all of us do every day.

All of us produce a certain number of cancer cells every day and we have the ability to kill a certain number of cancer cells every day as well. As long as we make fewer cancer cells than our ability to kill them, we will not develop cancer. Once the number of cancer cells reaches a certain number, it manifests clinically. Let us look at different scenarios. If you prefer, you can take a pen, paper, and even a simple calculator if you wish. I will use smaller numbers to make the calculation easy. In reality, these numbers are much higher.

Scenario #1: A normal person who does not develop cancer.

Let us assume that the number of new cancer cells produced per day is 50.

The ability of the normal person to kill cancer cells per day: 100.

As the 50 cancer cells are produced, the body's natural immunity kills those cells and the person will not develop cancer.

Scenario #2: A normal person who goes through a very stressful phase for a short period of time or a health condition with lowered immunity for a brief period of time.

Let us assume that the number of new cancer cells produced per day is 50.

The ability of the person to kill cancer cells per day goes down to 40 per day and every day the person adds 10 new cancer cells in the body increasing the burden of cancer cells in the body. This increases the number of new cells produced per day to 80 per day after a few days. Let us assume that after a few days, the person solves his stressful problem and his ability to kill cancer cells comes up to 100 cells per day. Now he is producing 80 new cancer cells per day and can kill 100 cancer cells per day, hence the burden of cancer cells will go down and he will not develop cancer.

Scenario #3: A normal person who goes through a very stressful phase for a prolonged period of stressful time or a health condition with lowered immunity.

Let us assume that the number of new cancer cells produced per day: 50.

The ability of the person to kill cancer cells per day goes down to 40 per day and every day the person adds 10 new cancer cells in the body increasing the burden of cancer cells in the body. This increases the number of new cells produced per day to 1000 per day after a few months. Let us assume that after a few months, the person solves his stressful problem and his ability to kill cancer cells comes up to 100 cells per day. Now he is producing 1000 new cancer cells per day and can kill only 100 cancer cells per day, hence the burden of cancer cells will keep on going up and once the number of cancer cells reaches a critical mass, he/she manifests cancer.

Scenario #4: A normal person who goes through a very stressful phase for a prolonged period of stressful time or a health condition with lowered immunity. After some time, he recovers from the stressful condition and increases his immunity by healthy lifestyle (diet, rest, adequate sleep, yoga, exercise, meditation):

Let us assume that the number of new cancer cells produced per day: 50

The ability of the person to kill cancer cells per day goes down to 40 per day and every day the person adds 10 new cancer cells in the body increasing the burden of cancer cells in the body. This increases the number of new cells produced per day to 1000 per day after a few months. Let us assume that after a few months, the person solves his stressful problem and his ability to kill cancer cells comes up to 100 cells per day. Now he changes his lifestyle with a vegetarian diet with almost 10 servings of fruits and vegetables per day, more rest, adequate sleep, regular yoga, regular exercise, regular meditation that increased his ability to kill cancer cells to 1100 per day. Now he is producing 1000 new cancer cells per day and he has increased his ability to kill cancer cells to 1100 per day, hence the burden of cancer cells will keep on going down every day and the person will not develop cancer.

The cancer cells are very strange and are difficult to understand. There are many known and unknown causes of cancer. This is my simplistic unproven view of the genesis of cancer.

In the mathematical way of surviving cancer also everything matters, be it a healthy diet, exercise, adequate sleep, adequate rest, regular meditation, regular prayers!

We all are born with the ability to kill a certain number of cancer cells every day.

We will discuss a few more different scenarios.

Scenario #5: A patient with early cancer becomes cancer-free after treatment with radiation, chemotherapy, or surgery: Let us assume that we can kill 100 cancer cells per day and let us assume a patient with cancer has 6000 cancer cells and produces 100 new cancer cells per day. Since cell growth occurs exponentially, this calculation is incorrect, but this helps make my point. This person's immunity will be able to keep cancer from growing by killing all the new cells every day without shrinking cancer.

If we can kill 3000 cancer cells by radiation, chemotherapy, or surgery, this person will have 3000 cancer cells left. Now he will make 75 new cancer cells every day and kill 100 cancer cells every day. In other words, the number of cancer cells will go down by 25 (100 cells killed minus 75 new cells produced equals 25 fewer cells per day) every day. On day #61, this patient will have no cancer cells left and he will be cancer-free!

Scenario #6: Intermediately advanced cancer treated with surgery alone:

Number of cells killed per day: 100

Number of cancer cells at the time of diagnosis: 15000

Number of cancer cells produced per day at the time of diagnosis: 250

Number of cancer cells killed by surgery: 3000

Number of cancer cells left after surgery: 12000

Number of new cancer cells produced per day after the surgery: 200

This patient's cancer will add 100 cells per day if her/his immunity kills 100 cells per day. This cancer will continue to grow despite surgery and hence may benefit from another strategy to eliminate cancer.

Scenario #7: Intermediately advanced cancer treated with surgery and chemotherapy:

Number of cancer cells killed per day: 100

Number of cancer cells at the time of diagnosis: 15000

Number of cells produced per day at the time diagnosis: 250

Number of cancer cells killed by surgery: 3000

Number of cancer cells left after surgery: 12000

Number of new cells produced per day after the surgery: 200

This patient's cancer will add 100 cells per day if her/his immunity kills 100 cells per day out of the 200 new cells produced. This cancer will continue to grow despite surgery.

Now, the doctor added chemotherapy and killed 3000 more cells leaving 9000 cells.

Number of new cancer cells per day after surgery and chemotherapy: 150

The person can kill 100 cells per day.

This person will continue to add 50 cells per day resulting in the growth of cancer despite surgery and chemotherapy.

Scenario #8: Intermediately advanced cancer treated with surgery, chemotherapy, and radiation:

Number of cancer cells killed per day: 100

Number of cancer cells at the time of diagnosis: 15000

Number of cancer cells produced per day at the time of diagnosis: 250

Number of cancer cells killed by surgery: 3000

Number of cancer cells left after surgery: 12000

Number of new cells produced per day after the surgery: 200

This patient's cancer will add 100 cells per day if her/his immunity kills 100 cells per day. This cancer will continue to grow despite surgery.

Now, the doctor added chemotherapy and killed 3000 more cells leaving 9000 cells.

Then the doctor added radiation therapy and killed 1500 more cells leaving 7500 cells.

Number of new cancer cells per day after surgery, chemotherapy, and radiation: 125

The person can kill 100 cells per day.

This person will continue to add 25 cells per day.

This person will continue to add 25 cells per day to 7500 cancer cells, resulting in the continued growth of cancer exponentially.

Scenario #9: Intermediately advanced cancer treated with surgery, chemotherapy, radiation plus anti-cancer lifestyle such as dietary modification and meditation:

Number of cancer cells killed per day: 100

Number of cancer cells at the time of diagnosis: 15000

Number of cancer cells produced per day at the time of diagnosis: 250

Number of cancer cells killed by surgery: 3000

Number of cancer cells left after surgery: 12000

Number of new cancer cells produced per day after the surgery: 200

This patient's cancer will add 100 cells per day if her/his immunity kills 100 cells per day. This cancer will continue to grow despite surgery.

Now, the doctor added chemotherapy and killed 3000 more cells leaving 9000 cells.

Then the doctor added radiation therapy and killed 1500 more cells leaving 7500 cells.

Number of new cancer cells per day after surgery, chemotherapy, and radiation: 125

The person can kill 100 cells per day.

Supposing, the doctor suggests an anticancer lifestyle including a special diet with a lot of antioxidants and less sugar (e.g., fresh vegetables and spices such as turmeric/curcumin, Boswellia, ginger, black pepper, etc.) and a guided meditation that increased the ability of the person to kill 30 more cancer cells per day.

Now, the person can kill 130 cells per day and he is producing 125 new cells per day. That means he/she is killing more cancer cells than he/she makes resulting in progressive shrinking of cancer eventually to eliminate it. As the remaining cancer cells reduce in number, the new cancer cells produced goes down, and the ability to kill 125 cancer cells per day continues resulting in exponential shrinking of cancer. But you need to continue a healthy lifestyle. This is the power of lifestyle change in cancer management. I cannot make an evidence-based claim on this. But it makes perfect scientific sense to me and I feel that this anticancer lifestyle happened to me.

Scenario # 10: Very advanced cancer treated with surgery, chemotherapy, radiation plus anticancer lifestyle including dietary modification and meditation:

Number of cells killed per day from immunity: 100

Number of cancer cells at the time of diagnosis: 60000

Number of cells produced per day at the time of diagnosis: 1000

Number of cells killed by surgery: 30000

Number of cancer cells left after surgery: 30000

Number of new cells produced per day after the surgery: 500

This patient's cancer will add 500 cells per day and her/his immunity kills 100 cells per day. This cancer will continue to grow despite surgery.

Now, the doctor added chemotherapy and killed 6000 more cells leaving 24000 cells.

Then the doctor added radiation therapy and killed 6000 more cells leaving 18000 cells.

Number of new cancer cells per day after surgery, chemotherapy, and radiation: 300

The person can kill 100 cells per day.

Supposing, the doctor suggests an anticancer lifestyle including a special diet with a lot of antioxidants and less sugar (e.g., fresh vegetables and spices such as turmeric/curcumin, Boswellia, ginger, black pepper, etc.) and meditation that increased the ability of the person to kill 30 more cancer cells per day. In other words, a person will make 300 new cells per day and kill only 130 cells per day, adding 170 new cells every day resulting in an exponential growth of cancer despite all the treatments provided including stronger chemotherapy and radiation along with lifestyle changes. In other words, if the initial tumor burden is high, no treatment might work.

In the very early stages, cancer might go away even without lifestyle changes. And if the cancer burden is somewhere in the middle, lifestyle changes (dietary changes, exercise, rest, sleep, meditation, etc.) might make a difference between becoming cancer-free vs not becoming cancer-free. For this reason, early treatment is better. Don't delay therapy, not even by a week if you can.

Now, let us look at a mathematical way of preventing cancer even if you are genetically prone to developing cancer. Again, everything matters, be it a healthy diet, exercise, adequate sleep, adequate rest, regular yoga, meditation, and regular prayers!

Again, back to basics! We all make a certain number of cancer cells every day and we can kill a certain number of cancer cells every day. As long as we make fewer cancer cells than our ability to kill them, we will not develop cancer. It is very common to see clustering of cancer patients in certain families and communities. Breast cancer is very common in Ashkenazic Jews. That is the reason that Angelina Jolie got both her breasts removed before she could develop cancer so she will not have any breast tissue left to develop cancer! Quite a radical approach! Nowadays many do this after she did it. I don't blame them. A study of 5,405 U.S. women with the common Ashkenazi Jewish mutation that increases carriers' risk of breast cancer, who were treated at the Mayo Clinic during the 1990s, found that 45 percent chose prophylactic mastectomy, like Angelina Jolie. Bilateral prophylactic mastectomy is not that common. But prophylactic mastectomy of the opposite breast after one develops cancer in one breast is quite common. In those who are genetically prone to develop cancer, if we can increase their ability to kill cancer cells by improving the cancer immunity with dietary/lifestyle changes and meditation, we may be able to prevent cancers. Please know that these are not scientifically confirmed and please check with your physician.

Bilateral prophylactic mastectomy can reduce the breast cancer risk by 90 percent and the surgical removal of the ovaries can reduce breast cancer risk by about 50 percent. Other options are to take such as tamoxifen or raloxifene and increase surveillance through regular screenings with mammograms and MRIs. We do not know if Ashkenazi Jews or those who have BRCA gene mutation can reduce the risk of breast cancer by dietary changes and meditation. But a study to test this theory would be worthwhile, especially for those not going for bilateral prophylactic mastectomy. We know that people with BRCA or PALB2 gene mutations have a higher-than-average chance of developing breast cancer, and are more likely to develop it at a younger age. Women with a BRCA1 or BRCA2 mutation can have a 45–65% chance of being diagnosed with breast cancer before age 70. The main fact to remember is that the risk of developing breast cancer is not 100% if one has these mutations. Thirty-five to 55% of these women do not develop breast cancer till they turn 70. *In other words, cancer is not destiny among those who have a genetic risk and every measure should be taken to reduce that risk.* We know from studies that meditation and lifestyle changes cause changes in the telomeres which change the way cell functions express and function. Dean Ornish and colleagues found changes in prostate gene expression in men undergoing an intensive nutrition and lifestyle intervention (low-fat, whole-foods, plant-based nutrition, stress management techniques, moderate exercise, and participation in psychosocial group support). Gene expression profiles were obtained from 30 participants, pairing RNA samples from control prostate needle biopsy taken before intervention to RNA from the same patient's three-month post-intervention prostate biopsy. Two-class paired analysis of global gene expression using significance analysis of microarrays detected 48 up-regulated and 453 down-regulated transcripts after the intervention. This supports the potential benefit of lifestyle changes in preventing cancer.

ii. Harmony among five elements and causation of cancer

When we look at nature, five elements provide the foundation for the entire physical world—space, air, fire, water, and earth. Ayurveda is an ancient Indian discipline of medicine that recognizes these elements as the building blocks of all material existence. These elements are present in the outside world and inside our body as well. We are part of nature.

- We nourish ourselves with foods that come from the 'earth', and eventually, our body returns to the earthly matter from which it came.

- 'Water' is our life-sustaining liquid, making up more than 70 percent of our total body mass.

- 'Air' gives movement to biological functions, feeds every cell with oxygen, and removes the carbon dioxide that the body generates and needs to expel.

- 'Fire' provides the body with heat and radiant energy; it also exists within all metabolic and chemical actions.

- 'Space' provides the other elements with an opportunity to interact in the ways we just mentioned.

Generally, it is not easy to find out the exact reason behind developing cancer. But, there is a lot of data on the association of certain factors and the prevalence of cancer.

Environment (Macrocosm)	Human Body (Microcosm)
Earth: Food, sugar, salt, medicines, infections, probiotics.	**Earth:** Skin, muscle, fat, bones, gene microbes.
Water: Water, sodas, non-carbonated drinks (with sugar/sweeteners/color), juice.	Water: Body fluids, secretions in the respiratory and gastrointestinal systems.
Air: Air, occupational exposure to dust, smoke, other toxins, radiation exposure.	**Air:** Air in the lungs and the intestines, oxygen, carbon dioxide, other 'gas' elements in the body, internal radiation.
Space: Spiritual space (friends, family, spiritual guide).	**Space:** Body space, spiritual space (friends, family, spiritual guide).
Fire: External fire, extremes of temperature, sunlight, moonlight.	**Fire:** Emotion and wake/sleep centers in the brain, thyroid gland, adrenal glands, digestive juices, energy units of the body such as ATP* and NADPH**.

*Adenosine Triphosphate
** The reduced form of nicotine adenine dinucleotide phosphoric acid

Table: Five Elements of the Universe (Environment/Macrocosm) surrounding the body that affects the health and the five elements of the human body (microcosm)

Every health problem is due to the derangement of one or more of the five main elements of the world. They are earth, air, water, fire, and ether (space). The universe (macrocosm) is made of these five elements.

Our body, microcosm, is also made of these five elements. There is mutual interaction of these five elements in the macrocosm and microcosm. The body constantly consumes these five elements from the universe. The earth element that the body consumes is solid food, the water element is the liquids we consume, the air element is the air we breathe, the fire element is the external stress we go through, and the 'ether' is the 'space' of family and friends we interact with. The five elements inside the body are solid tissues—the earth element, body fluids—the water element, gaseous elements—the air element, internal stress leading to the stress hormones and the related hormones, and the digestive juice and energy units—fire element, and finally, stress control centers in the brain—the internal ether/space element. All the health problems of the world including cancer can be traced to an imbalance in one or more of these five elements. According to Ayurveda, life or existence is not a rigid compartment, but a harmonious flow. Even the five elements of which the whole universe is made up are not tight compartments of defined objects. They flow into one another. These elements affect a person's emotions, personality, health, and response to treatment.

Cancer is also due to the imbalance of these five elements in the body. Understanding these subtle aspects and healing them with re-balancing the five elements and medical treatment is a way to deal with this potentially life-threatening disease.

Cancer is caused by the excessive growth of cells. This excessive growth happens from some triggers to the cells. This trigger could be something that promotes the growth of certain cells or a lack of something that inhibits the growth of these cells. This stimulus leads to the excessive growth of cells and that could be traced to one or more of the five elements.

Cancers known to be associated with underexposure or over-exposure to certain specific elements are mentioned here:

Earth elements include the food we consume (colon cancer is more common among those who eat meat and eggs), certain medicines such as hormones (e.g., estrogen consumption is known to increase the risk of breast cancer and ovarian cancers, testosterone could worsen prostate cancer), medicines that suppress immunity (there is a higher risk of malignancies in organ transplant recipients since they are on immuno-suppressant medications to prevent organ rejection) and chemotherapy medicines (patients who have been treated with chemotherapy are at higher risk of developing second cancer, leukemias, and lymphomas), certain infections such as hepatitis C that causes liver cancer, herpes simplex virus that causes cervical (lower part of the uterus) cancer, human immunodeficiency viral infection (HIV/AIDS) that is associated with Kaposi's sarcoma and certain lymphomas and others. There is a fear that excessive sugar consumption increases the risk of cancers. But this association is unclear, but we know that cancer cells have a high affinity for sugar. Certain genetic disorders such as familial polyposis are associated with a higher risk of cancers.

Water elements include drinking water, carbonated drinks, non-carbonated colored and sweetened drinks or juices with or without additives, alcohol, and others. Role of added sugar, sweeteners, food colors, and preservatives causing cancer remain uncertain and unproven. Obesity is associated with a higher risk of certain cancers.

Air elements include air with inhaled toxins such as dust, industrial wastes, asbestos that is associated with mesothelioma of the lungs, tobacco smoke in active or passive smokers that is associated with a higher risk of lung cancers, bladder cancer, colon cancers, and other cancers, occupational exposure to petroleum or smoke that is associated with lung cancers from inhalation, scrotal cancer in chimney sweepers due to exposure of the scrotal skin to smoke, etc.

Toxic **space** (also called **ether** in the spiritual and Ayurvedic literature) includes exposure to excessive ultraviolet rays from sun exposure, occupational radiation exposure, exposure to radiation as the treatment of cancer, radioactive iodine therapy for thyroid problems, radiation exposure from warfare, etc. Radiation is known to be associated with skin cancers, lymphomas, leukemias, bone cancers, and others and this was a common observation among the survivors of the Hiroshima and Nagasaki atomic bomb explosion.

Release of internal **fire** includes body toxins or hormones from the body due to stress and emotions related to our innate nature, friends, family, colleagues and other human beings and animals we deal with (the company we keep). The relationship of stress, emotions, yoga, meditation, and physical exercise to cancer is unclear even though cancer prevalence is lower among those who are more physically active.

Chapter Eight

Different Ways to Prevent Cancer

i. Lifestyle transformation to prevent cancer by influencing the five elements

T he following points and the subsequent paragraphs indicate the different problems affecting different elements associated with different cancers and possible solutions. These associations suggest many measures that can be incorporated into the lifestyle of a patient with cancer and anybody who wants to prevent cancer. Please know that this is not a complete list and it does not promise results. There are many other elements, especially gene defects associated with cancers and there are certain measures that can be taken if recommended by medical experts.

Problems involving the earth element with some association with cancer risk and their solutions:

1. Problem: Meat and eggs

Solution: Plant-based food

2. Problem: Sugars and sweeteners

Solution: Avoid sugars and sweeteners including sweets, deserts, sodas, drinks with sugars and sweeteners, donuts. Remember that juice also has a lot of sugar.

3. Problem: Excess salt

Solution: Reduce or avoid salt, replace with other tastes using lime/lemon, condiments, ginger, etc.

4. Problem: Medicines such as estrogen, testosterone, chemotherapy, immunosuppressive medicines used in transplant recipients, autoimmune diseases such as lupus, rheumatoid arthritis, psoriasis, ulcerative colitis, Crohn's disease, and other conditions.

Solution: Avoid or use caution with medicines such as estrogens and testosterone. Chemotherapy medicines and immunosuppressives have to be prescribed judiciously.

5. Problem: Genes

Solution: Genetic counseling, avoid consanguineous marriages (don't marry a relative).

Prophylactic mastectomy in those with BRCA genes. Frequent colonoscopy, polypectomy, and sometimes prophylactic colectomy in those with familial polyposis or ulcerative colitis.

6. Problem: Infections such as HIV, hepatitis C, Human papillomavirus (HPV)

Solution: Prevent infections such as HIV and hepatitis C by avoiding high-risk sexual behavior and recreational drug abuse; treat HIV and hepatitis C with medications if already acquired, prevent human papillomavirus (HPV) infection with the HPV vaccine.

The interventions that affect the remaining four elements include:

Water: Promoting healthy consumption of clean water and avoiding or limiting the intake of juice, alcohol, carbonated, and noncarbonated drinks.

Air: Managing the quality of air, including choosing where to live depending upon the quality of air, choosing where to work depending on the quality of air at work, wearing appropriate personal protective devices, avoiding active smoking, avoiding the company of smokers to avoid passive smoking, avoiding occupational risk factors, including carcinogens such as many chemicals, radioactive materials, and asbestos; avoiding environmental exposure, for instance to radon and UV radiation, and fine particulate matter.

Fire: Choosing regular study, contemplation and meditation to alter the response to stress in life, sleeping, and resting well.

Ether/space: Physical exercise, meditation, sleep, good company of friends and family, protecting the skin by regulating the exposure to sunlight and using appropriate sunscreens, genetic counseling before having children in certain situations. In the era of increasing conflicts, avoiding wars, especially nuclear wars is extremely important for preventing loss of lives and also to prevent cancers. Five to six years after the Hiroshima and Nagasaki bombings in World War II, the incidence of leukemia increased noticeably among survivors. After about a decade, there was a higher prevalence of thyroid, breast, lung, and other cancers among the survivors.

Everything adds up!

Drinking a good amount of water, around 50-60 ounces a day, is a good habit. Periodic fasting may bring some balance to the system. Fasting may induce autophagy, which may be good for health. Autophagy is the body's way of cleaning out damaged cells in the body in order to replace them with healthy cells. Whether autophagy protects against cancer is a matter of intense research. Healthy water consumption is important. A woman weighing 150 pounds (i.e., 68 kilograms) has about 75-85 pounds (34 to 38 kg) of water. Daily consumption of 50 ounces of water amounts to 1188 pounds of water per year. In other words, 75 pounds of water in the body gets 'mixed' with about 1200 pounds of water that is consumed every year. Similarly, if that person eats two pounds of food per day, that person's body contents are getting 'mixed' with 730 pounds of food every year. When it comes to air, the situation is still more staggering. Our body (made up of about 20 gallons or 75 liters of matter) gets 'mixed' with 833,183 gallons or 3,153,000 liters of air per year. Why am I giving all these numbers? It is because I want you to realize that a small amount of contamination like dust or cigarette smoke in the air that we breathe, a small amount of color or pesticide in the food, or a small amount of color or sugar or sweetener in liquids like sodas adds up to a lot over the years. Of all these, we know that smoking causes cancer of the lungs and some other organs. We also know that exposure of the skin to smoke for prolonged periods of time can cause skin cancer. Do pesticides in vegetables, hormones in milk and meat, sugars or sweeteners in sodas and other sweet drinks cause cancer? We don't know the answer. Knowing that I developed cancer for some reason that I do not know of, I have tried to make my lifestyle simple and safe. I consider it as the anticancer lifestyle for me. For that reason, I do not drink sodas or sweetened drinks. I do not smoke and I never smoked in the past. I have stopped eating chicken. I never ate beef or pork and I still don't eat it. I stopped eating eggs, fish, and seafood for 10 years after I had cancer. Since I don't feel well after consuming lentils due to my incontinence, I have started eating fish and eggs in moderation. But my diet is predominantly plant-based.

ii. Cancer prevention diet:

The principle behind a cancer diet or cancer prevention diet is creating a harmony of earth and water elements in the body (microcosm) and the universe (macrocosm). It is to be noted that these diets have not been subjected to rigorous trials that medicines go through. You can help me reach more people if you could leave an honest review at www.amazon.com and share this information with your friends and family.

'Cancer prevention happens in the kitchen.'

-Tricia Petzold MD, Salt lake city, Utah.

What we eat goes to our stomach, which is like the root of our system. Like a tree, which derives its nutrients and energy from its root system, humans derive their nutrients and energy from what is put into the stomach. From our stomach, our entire body is nourished. As the old saying goes, "You are what you eat." Finding the right diet, based on our constitution, is the first and foremost step in keeping your whole body healthy, youthful, and energetic.

In fact 'we are what we eat, drink, breathe, and think'. Our health is dictated by the environment that the body cells are immersed in. That environment consists of the food we eat, liquids that we drink, the air we breathe, and our 'mind/thought process' that affects the internal chemical/hormonal environment. This environment can often modify the response to the genetic signals in the body. You can help me reach more people if you could leave an honest review at www.amazon.com and share this information with your friends and family.

Healthy eating tips:

- Eat in moderation

- Follow 5-2-1-0 philosophy

- Emphasize fresh vegetables and fruits and eat a diet, which is mostly plant-based, locally grown, without using pesticides and growth hormones, preferably organic. Eat the locally grown, seasonal vegetables and fruits.

- Match your food with your personality: Educate yourself on proper nutrition, be sensitive to your body, and see what foods work for you. Match the type of food to the personality. Eat food that is moderate in taste, moderately cooked, and fresh. Avoid extremes of taste, pungent or putrid food.

- Eat as though you are feeding the 'God' in you:

- Eat with gratitude and a prayerful attitude. Pray if you wish before eating and express gratitude to your parents, teachers, friends, the person who cultivated the food, the person who cooked, and God/Infinity depending upon your beliefs.

- Eat food as an offering to God. Just like how you would not feed unhealthy food to God, don't feed unhealthy food to yourself. Before eating, ask yourself, 'would I feed this to God if I am given an opportunity?' If the answer is yes, go ahead and eat. If not, avoid that food.

- Buy organic if possible, especially for the 'dirty dozen' foods.

- Keep the 'chutneys' (these are certain spicy pastes and dressings in the Indian diet) and superfoods (cilantro, thyme, basil, turmeric, black pepper, ginger, etc.)

- Combine fruits and vegetables of different colors (remember rainbow). Different colored foods give different nutrients.

1. Whatever you eat, eat in moderation: In the holy *Song of God*, Chapter 6, verse 17, God uses the compound word *yuktahara-viharasya*, which means one who is moderate, restrained, and regulated in all activities. God states that such persons are eligible to practice *yoga*. Yoga means 'union with God', and not doing yoga asanas. Yoga means experiencing the divine God in you and around you.

God is stating that overeating and eating too little as well as extreme activity and complete inactivity are all detrimental to the union of individual consciousness with the ultimate consciousness (i.e., yoga). The same thing applies to excessive sleep and too little sleep as well as too much work which causes exhaustion. To that person who is disciplined in eating habits and exercise, who is regulated in sleep and waking, then union with the divine becomes easy and healthy living becomes a reality. This is integrating science, lifestyle and spirituality.

'*Moderation is adoration.*'—Nakta Venkata Raju, MD MRCP

2. 5-2-1-0 philosophy: Educate yourself on proper nutrition, be sensitive to your body, and see what foods work for you. 5-2-1-0 philosophy stands for five vegetables and fruits per day, less than two hours of recreational screen time per day (which refers to the use of smartphones, iPad, tablets, and computer screens for recreational purposes), at least one hour of physical activity for exercise every day, and no sugary drinks and sweets. This was designed for preventing and combating childhood obesity, but it is good for general health maintenance for adults as well. I was involved in promoting this movement to combat childhood obesity by educating the parents and school children in my volunteer role in the Texas Indo American Physicians Society and American Association of Physicians of Indian Origin with the help of my team members such as Drs Srini Potluri and Amit Guttigoli and Aradhana and Raj Asava of HungerMitao fame and many others.

Five stands for five vegetables and fruits in a day to provide fiber, antioxidants, vitamins, minerals, and some calories. Eating vegetables first reduces the need to eat other food materials. Some suggest that we increase this to 7–10 servings per day. If you are not a diabetic, it is easier to make this up by eating several fruits a day. One tennis ball size is considered one serving. One banana, one apple, or one medium-sized tomato is considered one serving each. I make a smoothie as mentioned earlier with two or more fruit servings (for example one banana and one apple), two servings of organic mixed leafy greens like spinach, kale, etc. along with a handful of nuts, some plant-based organic protein powder, and about more than half a liter (17 ounces) of water 6–7 days a week as a breakfast replacement. This gives me four servings or more right in the morning. It is a good idea to fill two-thirds of the plate with vegetables and eat it first. Please remember that potatoes, sweet potatoes, tapioca, and sweet corn are not considered vegetables. They are starch, considered as a source of carbohydrates.

'Two' stands for limiting the recreational screen time to less than two hours per day. This will reduce inactivity. This will give time to spend with family. In the craze of social media frenzy, it is very important to discipline our lives and limit the time we spend with smartphones, iPads, and television. This is as important to children as it is to adults all over the world. Between Facebook, WhatsApp, Snapchat, LinkedIn, Twitter, Instagram, Snapchat, and others, social media is rapidly consuming our lives. When we learned social etiquette during childhood, there were no social media.

We have to add this social media etiquette to our lives. Insisting on children not to use smartphones during family dinner time would be a reasonable starting point. One dangerous trend is using smartphones while driving. It is not only unhealthy but also dangerous. Tony Robbins, the motivational speaker and coach, recommends no screen time for two hours before going to bed.

'One' stands for at least one hour of physical activity every day. This increases the burning of calories. Physical activity can be a good mixture of light exercises like walking and strenuous exercises like running the treadmill and weight lifting. In the yoga world, we are taught to exercise using body weight as the weight. You can combine all these in a combination of your liking and convenience. If you want to be objective, take at least 6,000 steps in a day on average. If you are not wearing an Apple watch or iFit, most smartphones have a free 'Health' application that will count your steps. I use that every now and then to measure my level of activity. This may not be perfect, but there is no need to be perfect here. You can also simply walk for one hour every day. Think about doing these activities without playing music to the ears especially if you are walking outside.

'Zero' stands for avoiding sugary sodas, sugary beverages, and avoiding sweets. Generally, it is a good idea to be skeptical about anything which says '100%', 'natural', etc. From your own experience, if anything makes you hungry in two hours, that food is better avoided. Did you know that one can of soda of any brand has about 42 grams of sugar? That is as much sugar as most people would put in four to eight cups of tea depending upon how sweet-toothed you are! Did you know adding 100 calories (two-thirds of a can of regular soda) every day will make you gain 10 pounds in one year? That means if you are a soda drinker, just avoiding soda and sugary drinks will help you lose weight.

Adding nuts such as almonds, walnuts, and pecans, even ground-nuts/peanuts and cashews in your daily eating is a healthy habit. Go nuts! You can consume nuts as nuts, or in salad or curry or hummus. Did you know you can use almonds in place of coconut to prepare curry?

3. Emphasize on fresh vegetables and fruits and eat a diet that is mostly plant-based, locally grown, without using pesticides or hormones. Cut down or avoid meat. Have seasonal foods, preferably grown locally for the body to be in harmony with nature. This is one way to harmonize the five elements in your body (microcosm) with the five elements of the universe (macrocosm). Avoid canned food. Frozen food is reasonable but avoid it if possible. Avoid pre-cooked reheated food.

4. Match your food with your personality: More from my spiritual books to integrate lifestyle and navigating cancer! Match the different kinds of foods with similar kinds of personalities. In chapter 17 of the *Song of God*, God talks about three kinds of food, three kinds of offerings, and three kinds of characters. He talks about 'selfish and lazy (*tamasik*)', 'passionate (*rajasik*)', and 'peaceful (*saatvik*)' people. Lazy (*tamasik*) nature is that which fulfills one's desires, which are centered on the physical self. Passionate (*rajasik*) character aims at achieving one's ambitions and seeking material comfort. The peaceful (*saatvik*) character focuses on peace and noble thoughts and actions. In reality, the link between the kind of food and the character/nature of the person is mutual. The type of food affects the nature of the person and the people of certain nature eat their kind of food.

The *Song of God* recommends food in the mode of goodness (*saatvik*), probably vegetarian foods: "Foods dear to those in the mode of goodness increase the duration of life, purify one's existence, and give strength, health, happiness, and satisfaction." The Gita also says that such foods are "wholesome and pleasing to the heart." (BG 17.8)

At the same time, the same book says, "Foods that are too bitter, too sour, salty, hot, pungent, dry, and burning are dear to those in the mode of passion (*rajasik*). Such foods cause distress, misery, and disease." (BG 17.9)

And, it continues, "Food prepared more than three hours before being eaten, food that is tasteless, decomposed and putrid, and food consisting of remnants and untouchable things is dear to those in the mode of darkness" (BG 17.10). In modern science, the field of probiotics is gaining popularity. Probiotics are 'healthy germs'. Foods such as pickles, yogurt, and buttermilk are natural sources of probiotics. These are some 'putrid' foods that may be healthy and hence are exceptions to this teaching.

'Make eating a spiritual experience and a spiritual exercise. Feed yourself as though you are feeding God.'

5. Eat as though you are feeding the 'God' in you: Regardless of the food, eat with gratitude, a prayerful attitude, and mental poise. Pray before eating and eat with family without any TV or audio background. There is a common prayer from the *Song of God* (BG 4.24) recited before eating.

The English translation of that verse goes as follows:

The whole creation, being the gross projection of God, the Cosmic Consciousness itself; the food too is God, the process of offering it is God, it is being offered in the fire of God. He who thus sees that God in action reaches God alone. (BG:4:24)

The simpler interpretation and application of this verse is to prepare and eat food as an offering to God. Feed yourself as though you are feeding God. When you are feeding God, you are likely to choose only healthy food in a healthy proportion. The 14th verse of the 15th chapter of Gita is also commonly chanted before eating making eating a spiritual experience.

The *Song of God* (Gita) and several other scriptures teach us that our body is a temple. Considering food as an offering to God makes a lot of sense. It allows us to surrender to God before eating, but more important-ly, it allows us to express gratitude to the food, the people who cultivated food, the people who prepared food, the people who served food, and finally God for making the whole process possible. It also is an opportunity to sit together with family and friends and appreciate the divinity in the food and people involved in the food coming to our plates. This is very well practiced in the east and the west in all faiths. Sometimes I feel it is better practiced in the US by the Americans who grew up locally. This is a popular nursery rhyme:

"Thank you, God, for the world so sweet,

Thank you, God, for the food we eat,

Thank you, God, for the birds that sing,

Thank you, God, for everything.'

This sounds biblical, simple, and easy.

'We thank you, Lord, for giving us the food we need for living.

So bless us while we eat it because we really need it.'

'We thank you for the food, Lord. For Mom and Dad and you, Lord, the food, the fun, the friendship, of your big Family.' All these are exceptional, simple, and powerful. Pick one or all of them and practice every day. All these are ways to practice gratitude daily in our lives. If you are not doing it already, please try it yourself. You will love it.

6. Chew the food 21 times carefully and taste it deeply without rushing. Avoiding TV and other distractions while eating makes you eat slowly and generally, you end up eating less. Chewing well and eating slowly also reduces the glycemic index of food and that is healthier. If you want to be specific, I recently heard an expert suggest chewing the food 21 times before swallowing during the 'YOGACON21', a virtual conference of the American Association of Yoga and Meditation. Use this as a guide to consciously chew before gulping food.

7. Buy organic if possible: Buy organic apples, nectarines, eggs, spinach, and milk to minimize the intake of pesticides and hormones. Wash leafy vegetables well before cooking. Avocados, onions, oranges, pineapples, and bananas don't have many pesticides and hence they come in the 'clean fifteen'. If you want to be frugal, you don't have to buy organic 'clean dozen' fruits and vegetables. The recent list of 'dirty dozen' fruits and vegetables found to have the most pesticide residue by the Environmental Working Group includes strawberries, apples, nectarines, peaches, celery, grapes, cherries, spinach, tomatoes, sweet bell peppers, cherry tomatoes, and cucumbers. Buy these organic. Don't worry if you cannot afford organic fruits and vegetables. It is still a healthy practice to eat fruits and vegetables of any kind and all kinds. If you are going to buy sodas, sweets, and fried food, please divert that money to buy fruits and vegetables instead.

8. Keep the chutneys and the superfoods: Drink tea (four cups a day or four tea bags a day) and consume turmeric and tamarind. Mint, 'tulsi' (basil), cilantro, thyme, and other similar leaves are powerhouses of nutritious elements. These are superfoods. Don't eliminate them. Make fresh chutney (spiced herbal paste) out of them or use them in whatever way you want to. Readymade bottled chutney may not give all the benefits of fresh chutney. Spice up the tea! Add some ginger, cardamom, or cinnamon to your tea. Add some lemongrass to your tea. For coffee lovers, it is alright to have coffee in moderation. I heard it is good for the brain!

9. Combine fruits and vegetables of different colors: Different colors in fruits and vegetables give different nutrients. Remember the rainbow when buy them.

Have a healthy day filled with healthy food, tasty food, love, and gratitude.

Remember the prayer 'may all in this world be healthy' (*Lokah Samastah Sukhino Bhavantu*) and remember to recite it every day. I do it most of the days!

c. Meditation for healing and cancer prevention

Please remember that meditation is never the primary treatment of cancer. It is complementary!

Buddha was asked: "What have you gained from meditation?" He replied: "Nothing." "However," Buddha said, "let me tell you what I lost: anger, anxiety, depression, insecurity, fear of old age, and death." Buddhism is big on experiencing and being in 'Nothingness (*shoonya* state)'. *Shoonya* means zero.

I have used yoga, pranayama, and meditation as an adjunct in my treatment and for cancer prevention on my own. This is my cancer meditation or cancer prevention meditation without making any claims. Meditation is the delicate art of contemplating and letting go of all the efforts to relax into your true nature which is love, joy, peace, and 'Infinity'. Some would say that meditation is a conscious state of thinking nothing. Meditation is that which gives you deep rest. The rest in meditation is deeper than the deepest sleep that you can ever have. When the mind becomes free from agitation, is calm and serene and at peace, meditation 'happens'.

The benefits of meditation are diverse. It is an essential practice for mental hygiene. A calm mind, good concentration, clarity of perception, improvement in communication, blossoming of skills and talents, an unshakable inner strength, healing, the ability to connect to an inner source of energy, relaxation, and rejuvenation are all natural results of meditating regularly. In today's world where stress comes faster than the mind can perceive, meditation has become more of a necessity. To be unconditionally happy and to have peace of mind, we need to tap into the power of meditation.

Having gone through the emotional and physical experience of the diagnosis of cancer at the age of 41 years followed by chemotherapy, radiation, and surgery has given me first-hand experience with the suffering a cancer patient goes through and the fight that a cancer patient has to put forth. Being a physician has given me good insight into what goes on within the cancer cells and how chemotherapy, radiation, surgery, and other forms of therapy work.

These experiences, my interactions with my patients for over 30 years, my encounter with and/or study of various experts in the field have helped me understand how meditation can help in dealing with and healing from potentially a life-threatening illness. Please note that meditation, as far as the current understanding is concerned, is not a primary therapy for most serious illnesses, but it is an effective complementary therapy. I recommend you give yourself enough time to learn and then practice meditation regularly depending upon your schedule. My recommendation would be to spend at least 20 minutes of your time daily on meditating. Little more is better. Yoga experts say that you have to be 'yoga state' twenty four hours of the day, seven days a week.

Before you start, sit or lie down in a comfortable position. Avoid hurting any part of the body to achieve any specific posture. If a posture hurts, that is not a good posture to meditate. It is hard to meditate if you are in pain. Close your eyes, make a circle with your thumb and the tip of the index finger to indicate controlling the ego with your intellect within you, the 'manager' within you. The pointing index finger represents ego and the dominant thumb represents the intellect in you. The three other fingers that you stretch indicates your experience in wake, sleep and dream states that you will transcend to meditate. Face the hand and the remaining three fingers forward in front of your knees if you are sitting upright on the floor with crossed legs, upwards on your thighs if you prefer to sit on a chair with your feet touching the floor or upwards by the side of your body if you want to be lying down.

After you get better at meditation, go to the next level. Closer to the end of the meditation, focus on your forehead deep inside, and feel the bliss. I call this divine eye meditation. This is a deeper level of meditation. The divine eye is believed to be located in the forehead between the two visible eyes and farther inside your brain. Medically, I think that the 'divine eye' encompasses those parts of the brain which deal with emotions, endocrine regulation, and regulation of sleep. These parts in medical language are the frontal lobes, hypothalamus, reticular activating system, pineal body, and amygdala. Brain scans have shown increased activity in certain parts of the brain deep inside the forehead during deep meditation. The European Journal of Pain in 2005 published magnetoencephalography and functional magnetic resonance imaging of the brain of a yoga master who claimed not experiencing pain during deep meditation. Following a painful stimulus, they found less or no activity in parts of the brain that sense pain and increased activity in those parts of the brain (insula and cingular cortex), which mediate the emotional response to pain.

"The peace and love that we most often talk about and seek, we have within ourselves."

— Master Ching Hai.

Future is in our hands, so you can make it beautiful or you can make it worse, it's up to you. I mostly practiced meditation every day and still do it. I created a few techniques on my own. You can take help from them and enroll with a good teacher to learn. I have repeated the lines that have to be repeated during the meditation deliberately for you to get the real experience of meditation when you read this at the expense of adding pages to the book.

1. Good energy in and bad energy out breathing meditation (Modified Pranayama):

Sit comfortably and with your eyes closed, concentrate on the part of your forehead in between your eyes. Now concentrate deep inside your forehead and feel/imagine the brightness within you. As you feel the brightness, start focusing on your breathing. As I breathe in I invoke good energy flowing inside me through my nostrils via the forehead and as I breathe out I feel the bad energy flowing out of my body through my nostrils.

'Good energy flowing in as I inhale...'

Pause your breath for 5–12 seconds, pause... pause... pause... pause... pause... pause... pause

Bad energy flowing out as I exhale...

Pause... pause... pause... pause

'Good energy flowing in as I inhale ...'

Pause your breath for 5–12 seconds, pause... pause... pause... pause... pause... pause... pause

Bad energy flowing out as I exhale...

Pause... pause... pause... pause

'Good energy flowing in as I inhale...'

Pause your breath for 5–12 seconds, pause... pause... pause... pause... pause... pause

Bad energy flowing out as I exhale...

Pause... pause... pause... pause

(repeat this practice of 'Good energy flowing in as I inhale... pause... bad energy flowing out as I exhale...' nine more times)

Strength comes in as I inhale...

Pause...

Weakness going out as I exhale...

Pause...

Strength comes in as I inhale...

Pause...

Weakness going out as I exhale...

Pause...

Comfort comes in as I inhale...

Pause...

Pain going out as I exhale...

Pause...

Comfort comes in as I inhale...

Pause...

Pain going out as I exhale...

Pause...

Comfort comes in as I inhale...

Pause...

Pain going out as I exhale...

Pause...

Love coming in as I inhale...

Pause...

Hatred going out as I exhale...

Pause...

Love coming in ...

Pause...

Hatred going out...

Pause...

Love coming in as I inhale...

Pause...

Hatred going out as I exhale...

Pause...

Love coming in...

Pause...

Hatred going out ...

Pause...

Forgiveness coming in...

Pause...

Hatred going out....

Pause...

Forgiveness coming in ...

Pause...

Hatred going out...

Pause...

Blessings coming in...

Pause...

Negative thoughts flowing out...

Pause...

Blessings flowing in...

Pause...

Negative thoughts flowing out...

Pause...

... Pause for 5–12 seconds after you breathe in before you breathe out. As you practice, it becomes easier to pause your breath. As you pause your breath, feel the divine light inside your forehead, in between your eyebrows.

2. 'Cancer Healing Meditation' for people of all faiths:

In this meditation, you will be invoking God for healing. Please repeat after me in your mind. If you want, you may recite with me loudly so you can hear it. If you do not believe in God, replace 'God' with the term 'Infinity'.

I invoke God to remove all the obstacles in my journey of treatment of this cancer.

I invoke God to remove all the obstacles in my journey of prevention of recurrence of cancer.

I invoke God to remove all the obstacles in my journey of healing the body from the ravages of the disease and the treatment.

Deep breath in, pause... deep breath out, pause... (breathe in and breathe out three times)

I invoke God for the wealth of knowledge and wisdom in choosing the right place and the right doctor to get the best treatment from.

I invoke God for the wealth of knowledge and wisdom in choosing the right treatment options available to me.

I invoke God for the wealth of knowledge and wisdom in knowing my disease and its impact on myself, my family members, and my friends.

Deep breath in, pause... deep breath out, pause... (breathe in and breathe out three times)

I invoke God for the wealth of resources needed to take the best treatment available without compromising supporting my family

Deep breath in, pause ... deep breath out, pause... (breathe in and breathe out three times)

I invoke God for the healing from cancer and from the side effects of treatment of cancer.

I invoke God to keep my emotions under control during days or moments that may be turbulent for me and for people who care for me. I understand that when I am unwell, it is not just affecting me alone, but my whole family, biological and non-biological, is affected. Give me the ability to comfort them. Give us the ability to help each other.

I invoke God to flow in the good air that I breathe (~5-10 second pause between a deep breath in and a deep breath out).

I invoke God to flow into my body in the chemotherapy medicines to restore my health.

I invoke God to get into the radiation machine to restore my health.

I invoke God to get into my surgeon's knife to restore good health and to remove the unwanted tissue that does not belong to me.

Deep breath in, pause... deep breath out, pause ... (three times)

I invoke God who is the epitome of strength, loyalty, and humility.

I invoke God for the strength to endure the pain, nausea, and other discomforts from the disease and the treatment.

I invoke God for the medicines from heaven to bring me back to life.

Deep breath in, pause... deep breath out, pause... (breathe in and breathe out three times)

I invoke God to kill all the cancer cells in my body

I invoke God not to let any cancer cells spill to any organs.

I invoke God's multi-pronged attack on the cancer cells to eliminate them at all stages of development.

I invoke God's tongue to lick away all the remaining cancer cells.

I invoke God's lotus to soothe my injured areas and relieve them from suffering.

I invoke God's blessings from Her/His hands and the eyes.

I invoke God's blessings from Her/His hands and the eyes.

I invoke God's blessings from Her/His hands and the eyes.

I invoke God's halo of protection around my head.

I invoke God's halo of protection around my head.

I invoke God's halo of protection around my head.

I invoke God's halo of protection all around me.

I invoke God's halo of protection all around me.

I invoke God's halo of protection all around me.

Deep breath in, pause... deep breath out, pause... (three times)

3. Healing vibrations from OM

Start with expressing gratitude to your mentors (Gurus) in your own way (Om Gurubhyo Namaha).

In this meditation, you will recite Om. Om actually is A, U, M. This is supposed to create healing vibrations in the body. Even though OM is quoted in a lot of Hindu scriptures, you do not have to be a Hindu to practice this meditation. OM is also sacred for other religions that originated in India such as Sikhism, Buddhism, and Jainism. Some believe that OM is part of Amen, Amin, and Shalom which are Christian, Islam, and Jewish expressions of divinity respectively. Irrespective of your religious beliefs I believe it is a good practice to salute your Guru in the beginning and express gratitude.

In OM or AUM, 'A' stands for the wakeful state, 'U' stands for the dream state, 'M' stands for sleep state and the silence after 'M' stands for 'Infinity', the unmanifest state of the pure self. Transcend the self, manifesting in the wake, dream, and sleep states and merge into Infinity with this meditation.

Keep the room silent without TV, radio, or any music.

Shut off the lights.

Sit upright with crossed legs or some comfortable position.

Make a circle with the tip of your index finger representing ego and the tip of your thumb representing the 'Master' and keep both hands on your knees with the palms facing upwards.

Close your eyes.

Repeat after me.

Take a deep breath in.

Pause... pause... pause... pause...

As you breathe out chant Oooommmmmm...

Pause... feel the light inside your forehead, feel the divinity, feel the light, feel the love, feel the peace, feel your true state of pure consciousness, feel the ONENESS WITH THE UNIVERSE, feel the all-loving, all-compassionate, all-powerful, fearless, birthless, deathless, all-pervading, self-effulgent, complete, ONE without a second, witness consciousness, pure consciousness, feel the INFINITY (5–12 seconds)

Take a deep breath in.

Pause... pause... pause... pause...

As you breathe out chant Oooommmmmm

Pause... feel the light inside your forehead, feel the divinity, feel the light, feel the love, feel the peace, feel your true state of pure consciousness, feel the ONENESS WITH THE UNIVERSE, feel the all-loving, all-compassionate, all-powerful, fearless, birthless, deathless, all-pervading, self-effulgent, complete, ONE without a second, witness consciousness, pure consciousness, feel the INFINITY (5–12 seconds)

Take a deep breath in

Pause... pause... pause... pause...

As you breathe out chant Oooommmmmm

Pause... (5–12 seconds)

Take a deep breath in

Pause... pause... pause... pause...

As you breathe out chant Oooommmmmm

Pause... (5–12 seconds)

Take a deep breath in

Pause... pause... pause... pause...

As you breathe out chant Oooommmmmm

Pause... feel the light inside your forehead, feel the divinity, feel the light, feel the love, feel the peace, feel your true state of pure consciousness, feel the ONENESS WITH THE UNIVERSE, feel the all-loving, all-compassionate, all-powerful, fearless, birthless, deathless, all-pervading, self-effulgent, complete, ONE without a second, witness consciousness, pure consciousness, feel the INFINITY (5–12 seconds)

Take a deep breath in

Pause... pause... pause... pause...

As you breathe out chant Oooommmmmm

Pause... feel the light inside your forehead, feel the divinity, feel the light, feel the love, feel the peace, feel your true state of pure consciousness, feel the ONENESS WITH THE UNIVERSE, feel the all-loving, all-compassionate, all-powerful, fearless, birthless, deathless, all-pervading, self-effulgent, complete, ONE without a second, witness consciousness, pure consciousness, feel the INFINITY (5–12 seconds)

Take a deep breath in

Pause... pause... pause... pause...

As you breathe out chant Oooommmmmm

Pause... (5–12 seconds)

Take a deep breath in

Pause... pause... pause... pause...

As you breathe out chant Oooommmmmm

Pause... (5–12 seconds)

Take a deep breath in

Pause... pause... pause... pause...

As you breathe out chant Oooommmmmm

Pause... feel the light inside your forehead, feel the divinity, feel the light, feel the love, feel the peace, feel your true state of pure consciousness, feel the ONENESS WITH THE UNIVERSE, feel the all-loving, all compassionate, all-powerful, fearless, birthless, deathless, all-pervading, self-effulgent, complete, ONE without a second, witness consciousness, pure consciousness, feel the INFINITY (5–12 seconds)

Take a deep breath in

Pause... pause... pause... pause...

As you breathe out chant Oooommmmmm

Pause... (5–12 seconds)

Take a deep breath in

Pause... pause... pause... pause...

As you breathe out chant Oooommmmmm

Pause... (5–12 seconds)

Take a deep breath in

Pause... pause... pause... pause...

As you breathe out chant Oooommmmmm

Pause... feel the light inside your forehead, feel the divinity, feel the light, feel the love, feel the peace, feel your true state of pure consciousness, feel the ONENESS WITH THE UNIVERSE, feel the all-loving, all-compassionate, all-powerful, fearless, birthless, deathless, all-pervading, self-effulgent, complete, ONE without a second, witness consciousness, pure consciousness, feel the INFINITY (5–12 seconds)

Take a deep breath in

Pause... pause... pause... pause...

As you breathe out chant Oooommmmmm

Pause... (5–12 seconds)

Take a deep breath in

Pause... pause... pause... pause...

As you breathe out chant Oooommmmmm

Pause... (5–12 seconds)

Take a deep breath in

Pause... pause... pause... pause...

As you breathe out chant Oooommmmmm

Pause... feel the light inside your forehead, feel the divinity, feel the light, feel the love, feel the peace, feel your true state of pure consciousness, feel the ONENESS WITH THE UNIVERSE, feel the all-loving, all-compassionate, all-powerful, fearless, birthless, deathless, all-pervading, self-effulgent, complete, ONE without a second, witness consciousness, pure consciousness, feel the INFINITY (5–12 seconds)

Take a deep breath in

Pause... pause... pause... pause...

As you breathe out chant Oooommmmmm

Pause... (5–12 seconds)

Take a deep breath in

Pause... pause... pause... pause...

As you breathe out chant Oooommmmmm

Pause... (5–12 seconds)

Take a deep breath in

Pause... pause... pause... pause...

As you breathe out chant Oooommmmmm

Pause... feel the light inside your forehead, feel the divinity, feel the light, feel the love, feel the peace, feel your true state of pure consciousness, feel the ONENESS WITH THE UNIVERSE, feel the all-loving, all-compassionate, all-powerful, fearless, birthless, deathless, all-pervading, self-effulgent, complete, ONE without a second, witness consciousness, pure consciousness, feel the INFINITY (5–12 seconds)

Take a deep breath in

Pause... pause... pause... pause...

As you breathe out chant Oooommmmmm

Pause... feel the light inside your forehead, feel the divinity, feel the light, feel the love, feel the peace, feel your true state of pure consciousness, feel the ONENESS WITH THE UNIVERSE, feel the all-loving, all-compassionate, all-powerful, fearless, birthless, deathless, all-pervading, self-effulgent, complete, ONE without a second, witness consciousness, pure consciousness, feel the INFINITY (5–12 seconds)

Take a deep breath in

Pause... pause... pause... pause...

As you breathe out chant Oooommmmmm

Pause... feel the light inside your forehead, feel the divinity, feel the light, feel the love, feel the peace, feel your true state of pure consciousness, feel the ONENESS WITH THE UNIVERSE, feel the all-loving, all-compassionate, all-powerful, fearless, birthless, deathless, all-pervading, self-effulgent, complete, ONE without a second, witness consciousness, pure consciousness, feel the INFINITY (5–12 seconds)

Take a deep breath in

Pause... pause... pause... pause...

As you breathe out chant Oooommmmmm

Pause... feel the light inside your forehead, feel the divinity, feel the light, feel the love, feel the peace, feel your true state of pure consciousness, feel the ONENESS WITH THE UNIVERSE, feel the all-loving, all-compassionate, all-powerful, fearless, birthless, deathless, all-pervading, self-effulgent, complete, ONE without a second, witness consciousness, pure consciousness, feel the INFINITY (5–12 seconds)

... Slowly open your eyes.

4. Cancer healing meditation for Hindus

(Hindus might appreciate this better. If you are not a Hindu you can skip this meditation. However, you are welcome to do this.)

Chant OM as you breathe out. Each Om should be in one breath lasting for approximately five seconds with about four seconds pause between each Om. As you practice, the pause will get longer and longer.

In this meditation, you will be invoking God with name and form for healing. Invoking God in name and form can be an extremely powerful and easier way of meditation using visualization and sound. It is a privilege to experience the formless God in form and names. Please repeat after me in your mind. If you want you may recite with me loudly as you read this so you can hear it. Please feel free to use deities of your preference depending upon how you feel connected.

I salute my teachers and Gurus for guiding me in different ways.

Om Shri Gurubhyo Namaha

Om Shri Gurubhyo Namaha

Om Shri Gurubhyo Namaha

I invoke Lord Ganesha to remove all the obstacles in my journey of treatment of this cancer.

I invoke Lord Ganesha to remove all the obstacles in my journey of prevention of recurrence of cancer.

I invoke Lord Ganesha to remove all the obstacles in my journey of healing my body from the ravages of the disease and the treatment.

Om Shri Ganeshaaya Namaha

Om Shri Ganeshaaya Namaha

Om Shri Ganeshaaya Namaha

I invoke Goddess Saraswathi (also spelled as Saraswati) for the wealth of knowledge and wisdom in choosing the right place and the right doctor to get the best treatment from.

I invoke Goddess Saraswathi for the wealth of knowledge and wisdom in choosing the right treatment options available to me.

I invoke Goddess Saraswathi for the wealth of knowledge and wisdom in knowing my disease and its impact on myself, my family members, and my friends.

Om Shri Maha Saraswathyei Namaha

Om Shri Maha Saraswathyei Namaha

Om Shri Maha Saraswathyei Namaha

I invoke Goddess Laxmi for the wealth of resources needed to take the best treatment available without compromising supporting my family.

I invoke Goddess Laxmi for the wealth of resources needed to take the best treatment available without compromising supporting my family.

I invoke Goddess Laxmi for the wealth of resources needed to take the best treatment available without compromising supporting my family.

Om Shri Mahalaxmyei Namaha

Om Shri Mahalaxmyei Namaha

Om Shri Mahalaxmyei Namaha

I invoke Lord Vishnu for the healing from cancer and from the side effects of treatment of cancer treatment.

I invoke Lord Vishnu for the healing from cancer and from the side effects of treatment of cancer treatment.

I invoke Lord Vishnu for the healing from cancer and from the side effects of treatment of cancer treatment.

I invoke Lord Vishnu to keep my emotions under control during days or moments that may be turbulent for me and for people who care for me. I understand that when I am unwell, it is not affecting me alone, but my whole biological and non-biological family is affected. Give me the ability and courage to comfort them. Give us the ability to help each other.

I invoke Lord Vishnu to flow in the good air that I breathe (~10-second pause for a deep breath in and out).

I invoke Lord Vishnu to flow into my body in the chemotherapy medicines to restore health.

I invoke Lord Vishnu to get into the radiation machine to restore my health.

I invoke Lord Vishnu to get into my surgeon's knife to restore good health and to remove the unwanted tissue that does not belong to me.

Om Shri Maha Vishnave Namaha

Om Shri Maha Vishnave Namaha

Om Shri Maha Vishnave Namaha

I invoke Lord Hanuman who is the epitome of strength, loyalty, healing, and humility.

I invoke Lord Hanuman for the strength to endure the pain, nausea, and other discomforts from the disease and the treatment.

I invoke Lord Hanuman for Sanjivini, the same medicine that you brought from the mountains (Dronagiri, Meru, Himalayas) to bring Laxmana back to life.

I invoke Lord Hanuman for your humility, strength, fearlessness, loyalty, and Infinity

OM Shri Aanjaneyaayei Namaha

OM Shri Aanjaneyaayei Namaha

OM Shri Aanjaneyaayei Namaha

I invoke Lord Shiva for giving me the courage to conquer the fear of death

I invoke Lord Shiva to burn cancer cells into ashes

I invoke Lord Shiva's trident (Trishul) to kill the cancer cells

Om Namaha Shivaaya

Om Namaha Shivaaya

Om Namaha Shivaaya

I invoke Goddess Durga to kill all the cancer cells in my body

I invoke Goddess Durga (Kaali) not to let any cancer cells spill to any organs, just like you eliminated Rakhthabheejasura.

I invoke Goddess Durga's sword, the Chakra, the three-pronged Trishul, the mace, and other weapons to put forth a multi-pronged attack on the cancer cells to eliminate them at all stages of development.

I invoke Goddess Kaali's tongue to lick away all the remaining cancer cells.

I invoke Goddess Durga's lotus to soothe my injured areas and relieve them from pain and suffering.

I invoke Goddess Durga's blessings from Her hands and the eyes.

I invoke Goddess Durga's blessings from Her hands and the eyes.

I invoke Goddess Durga's blessings from Her hands and the eyes.

I invoke Goddess Durga's halo of protection inside my forehead.

I invoke Goddess Durga's halo of protection inside my forehead.

I invoke Goddess Durga's halo of protection inside my forehead.

I invoke Goddess Durga's halo of protection all around me.

I invoke Goddess Durga's halo of protection all around me.

I invoke Goddess Durga's halo of protection all around me.

Om Shri Durgaayei Namaha

Om Shri Durgaayei Namaha

Om Shri Durgaayei Namaha

5. Sudarshan Kriya Yoga and Inner Engineering:

I have learned Sudarshan Kriya, a powerful meditation technique that keeps our body and mind healthy. It is taught by The Art of Living Foundation, a non-profit, educational, and humanitarian organization operating in over 150 countries. The Art of Living Foundation was founded in 1981 by the world-renowned humanitarian and spiritual leader Sri Ravi Shankar. I was fortunate to learn it directly from him.

The Art of Living is more of a principle, a philosophy of living life to its fullest. It is more of a movement than an organization. Its core value is to find peace within oneself and to unite people in our society—people of different cultures, traditions, religions, and nationalities—thus reminding us all that we have one goal: to uplift human life everywhere.

It offers numerous highly effective educational and self-development programs, including breathing techniques, meditation, yoga, and practical wisdom for daily living, which have helped millions around the world completely transform their lives. It has helped many prisoners, war veterans, students, and regular people all over the world.

If you are looking forward to learning meditation, yoga, and pranayama, you can experience the Art of Living flagship course, THE HAPPINESS PROGRAM. The program is based on breathing techniques, authentic yoga, and effortless meditation.

Our breath is the bridge between the body and mind, and if we learn these breathing techniques, we can have a major say in our emotions, mind, and body. The Sudarshan Kriya taught in the program is an excellent technique to boost the immune system, overcome depression and recover from various health issues. Sudarshan Kriya elevates the life force (*prana*) and elevates our lives.

After the Happiness Program, there are more advanced courses where one experiences bliss in silence, gets to know oneself better, and basks in the glory of Self. Apart from advanced meditation programs, there are various other programs for different walks of life. I have only attended 'The Happiness Program' and practiced some variations of Sudarshan Kriya.

For more details on the benefit of Sudarshan Kriya, visit the link: http s://www.artofliving.org/in-en/what-sudarshan-kriya

More recently, I have attended the 'Inner Engineering' course by Sadhguru Jaggi Vasudev and I have been doing 'Shambhavi Kriya' most of the days since. This time again, I was fortunate to learn it from the 'Infinity' of inner engineering, Sadhguru himself. I attended it out of curiosity to know what it was since I have been conducting educational programs for the Texas Medical Association on the medical applications of yoga and meditation since 2014. I learned it, practiced it, and experienced it. Shambhavi Kriya is preceded by a few yoga asanas (postures) and consists of a series of breathing maneuvers, which come under the category of pranayama, meditation, and chanting. I have found it extremely helpful and I would recommend it to you as well. It is money and time well spent. I don't know if there is something special about Shambhavi Kriya and inner engineering. But my personal experience was something different, more than what I expected and it was something special. It is also possible that I am older now, I may have matured in the practice of yoga and meditation; it is possible that I was ready to experience it. I want to believe that this was inner engineering helping me experience 'Infinity'. It was indeed a transcendental experience. Interesting thing is that Sadhguru does not claim ownership to inner engineering or the Shambhavi Kriya that he teaches. He claims that inner engineering is very scientific and is accessible to all of us. Based on my own reading, scientific research supports that yoga and meditation improve an individual's health.

Most of the research that I have studied is on Transcendental Meditation, Mindfulness-Based Stress Reduction, and Sudarshan Kriya. You will find some useful scientific publications in pubmed.gov if you search under authors Orme-Johnson, David W, and Alexander C.N. You will find some publications showing improved cognitive flexibility, increased longevity, and decreased anxiety among the practitioners of Transcendental Meditation. There are also publications showing alteration in the steroid levels, slower progression of human immunodeficiency virus infection, decrease in the blood pressure, decrease in pain, and better control of thoughts in subjects who meditate. But I have a different and better personal experience with inner engineering and Shambhavi Kriya taught directly by Sadhguru than other meditation techniques. Despite my personal experience, I feel that I am not qualified enough to recommend any one of these techniques more than the others. I think the science of inner engineering is part of all these methods.

I prefer a technique for experiencing 'Infinity/Brahman' as in techniques based on non-duality (Advaita Vedanta based techniques) than Buddhist techniques of experiencing 'the state of nothing (*shoonya*)'. I think that 'Infinity'-based methods are relaxing, blissful, life-enhancing and empowering, and positive compared to Buddhist meditations which are mainly relaxing. There is nothing bad about any of these different methods and there is overlap between them. My suggestion to you is to explore and learn different techniques and adapt to the one you feel blissful with. Training is available in most parts of the world. Some cost more than others. All the organizations need funds to run their organizations, they all raise funds in different ways. Some rely on donations and some collect them directly from the direct beneficiaries. I am fine with both approaches. There are plenty of videos on YouTube. I prefer personal experience with a trained person. Feel free to explore and experience. When you are ready, you will find the right resource and the right teacher. Sometimes, you will find that the teacher will come to you instead of you going to the teacher.

"Learn to meditate from a qualified person and practice regularly in any way that you feel comfortable with and feel connected to"

iv. Visualization

Visualization aids a lot in healing in certain individuals. It is said that whatever you intend is what you get. I would visualize getting out of cancer by fighting the cancer cells and reducing them to melt away. I would further visualize getting back to normalcy and living a healthy and contented life with my family and friends. The meditation I have mentioned above where I would visualize the Divine taking over and saving me proved to be of great help to relax, rejuvenate, and empower me.

Soft music can help you to get into more soothing thoughts or you can take help from a guided meditation practitioner. The more strength you have inside, the better it is to fight the cancer cells and get well soon. The visualization is a powerful tool to receive the much-needed strength.

The 'consciousness' is very powerful. The baby develops from one cell to a complete human being. It knows where to develop which body part to what extent. When a cell can multiply itself and turn into a fully grown individual, then it can heal itself too when it loses its rhythm or some life-taking disease challenges you. Life is a combination of free will and destiny. If we imagine ourselves to be full of joy, love, and enthusiasm, the mind will get the strength to fight the side effects of chemotherapy and heal the body better.

One more powerful technique is to imagine the body part which has got cancer to be free from any disparities. Imagine it to be completely unblemished, healthy, and functioning properly.

The mind and whatever the mind is connected to in the immune system has the power to heal and acknowledging the body-mind connection will be beneficial.

v. Music and dancing for bliss and healing

Listening to music is a useful therapy for cancer patients to reduce anxiety, relax deeply, improve their sleep, diminish stress levels and release disturbing emotions. I listen and sing devotional songs in praise of God almost every day. The *bhajans* uplift my spirit and fill me with energy. I sing and chant prayers on deities such as God Hanuman and Goddess Durga who epitomize strength and healing. This is a personal choice and you can do this if you prefer and customize it to your faith, belief, and comfort level. Dancing and singing also help to elevate the mood and may make you feel joyful and experience Infinity. Some saints like Swami Ganapati Sacchidananda conduct healing music concerts and he has many CDs on healing music that he has sung. Some combine singing and dancing.

The devotees at ISKON (International Society of Krishna Consciousness) temples sing and dance for a good length of time. The founder of ISKON, His Holiness AC Prabhupada, apparently used to chant a holy verse 1008 X 18 times in one sitting. He taught classes on Vedic from India, which he claimed could affect the consciousness of a world afflicted with rampant materialism. He was a follower of the tradition of devotion (bhakti, love towards God) as the path to divine experience of Krishna Consciousness. He taught the holy verse *'Hare Rama Hare Rama Rama Rama Hare Hare, Hare Krishna Hare Krishna Krishna Krishna Hare Hare'*. The devotees call it the 'maha mantra', which means 'great mantra'. When you chant a holy word or sentence for a long period of time with utmost faith towards God, you experience bliss and can go into ecstasy.

This can be healing and this can be enlightening. I have done meditation and I have chanted this mantra, but I have not chanted it 18,144 times at a stretch. For that reason, I do not have first-hand experience with this. But I have experienced glimpses of bliss while doing meditation. This state of bliss gives you access to cosmic intelligence and that is what I call experiencing 'Infinity'. This experience is available to all of us in this life, right now. We can experience this 'out of the body experience' when we are deeply engrossed in what we do. It is not limited to traditional meditators. It can happen while reading a book, or singing, or playing a musical instrument, or dancing, or even while playing sports. If cancer in me were not to respond to treatment and every other thing I had done, I was planning to go to Dallas ISKON temple and chant the 'great mantra' 18,144 times regularly. I was hoping that it would take me to a different plane of existence, a different level of cosmic energy, and a different degree of immunity to heal my cancer. I do no know if that would have helped, but I believe it would. I am happy that I am better. Sage Patanjali, the author of '*Yoga Sutras*' (aphorisms on yoga) prescribes in one of the apho-risms to do anything regularly ('*nairantarya*') and for a prolonged period (*dheerga kaala*) to experience a bliss (yoga) state. Yoga state is a state of bliss. Dancing was never my thing. Doing any practice regularly for a prolonged period helps develop any habit, including doing exercise. Apparently, it takes around 66 days to develop a habit, some say less and some say more. I think the truth is that it depends upon the person and what one person is practicing. Once you keep doing the same thing, at the same time, every day for a few months (for example, 66 days) it becomes a routine, you get good at it and it becomes easy to continue.

'Practicing anything like meditation or exercise every day at the same time for a prolonged period for over ~66 days helps you make it a habit.' --*Source Unknown (my source is Sunil Tulsiani)*

Apparently, when Swami Prabhupada, the founder of ISKCON came to the US, he started an office in the ghettos of New York and taught his followers chanting the mantra 18,144 times a day, every day. Some of them experienced the state of ecstasy and felt that the experience was similar to what they would experience when they took recreational drugs like cocaine and/or 'Ecstasy'. It helped some people quit abusing drugs. But it also attracted more people who used recreational drugs and created some controversy. But the great sage Swami Prabhupada took that risk to develop the organization. Today, ISKCON has grown to be the organization that is the source of the Bhagavad Gita to the maximum number of families in the world. ISKCON has grown to be the organization that is the source of the ecstatic experience of 'Krishna Consciousness'/'Infinity' to thousands of families in the world.

What did I do?

I love to sing. I don't dance. I do not know any classical music. But we sang devotional songs every day as a family before dinner when I was growing up. I still know many of those songs, and I have learned a few more devotional songs since then. I sing or at least listen to some devotional songs every day. I find a lot of strength in singing some of these, especially those about God manifesting as deities representing healing and strength. I feel this is one of the ways of unveiling the Infinity within me and experiencing the infinite healing strength within me. I am coming back to non-duality! But, believe me, that is very powerful. My mother loved to sing, but in 2020 she developed a minor stroke due to which she was unable to say the correct words. I used to sing to her often when I talked to her till her body left this world in April 2021 from a massive stroke. Without being an expert, I either give spiritual discourses or listen to them in small groups of friends most days. Thanks to YouTube, I have listened to thousands of spiritual discourses. My friends Raju and Gopal created a virtual platform about 15 years ago, and I have continued to participate in these activities. That has been my way of learning. This is also my way of spending about 90 minutes in the restroom every day when I give myself an enema! I use these opportunities to sing as well. A lot of singing and reading happens in my restroom!

vi. Exercise for prevention and treatment of cancer

Exercise plays a crucial role in recovering from cancer. Meyerhardt and coworkers in 2006 and Friedenreich and coworkers in 2016 have shown that increased physical activity has been associated with a reduction in mortality in survivors of colorectal cancer. This may be explained by exercise-induced changes in systemic pathways. In the Journal of Physiology (J Physiol. 2019 Apr;597(8):2177–2184. DOI: 10.1113 /JP277648. Epub 2019 Mar 20.) Devin and coworkers showed that short bursts of high-intensity exercise (4 X 4 minutes at 85-95% peak heart rate) reduced the colon cancer cell number in the laboratory and increased the inflammatory cytokines (interleukin-6 and tumor necrosis factor) immediately following exercise. Based on many other studies Ashcroft and co-workers suggested that exercise be an adjunct therapy for cancer (Semin Radiat Oncol. 2019 Jan;29(1):16–24. DOI: 10.1016/j.semradonc.2018.10.001).

The following information is a summary of the role of exercise in different cancers from the website of the National Cancer Institute at

Bladder cancer: In large studies, bladder cancer was 13–15% less common among those who exercise.

Breast cancer: In a large study in 2016, the most physically active women had a 12–21% lower risk of breast cancer than those who were least physically active.

Colon cancer: In a 2016 meta-analysis of 126 studies, individuals who engaged in the highest level of physical activity had a 19% lower risk of colon cancer than those who were the least physically active.

Endometrial cancer: In a meta-analysis of 33 studies, highly physically active women had a 20% lower risk of endometrial cancer than women with low levels of physical activity. Obesity is a strong risk factor for endometrial cancer.

Esophageal cancer: In large studies, it has been found that the individuals who were most physically active had a 21% lower risk of esophageal cancer than those who were least physically active.

Kidney (renal cell) cancer: An analysis of over one million individuals found that leisure-time physical activity was linked to a 23% reduced risk of kidney cancer.

Stomach (gastric) cancer: A 2016 study reported that individuals who were most physically active had a 19% lower risk of stomach cancer than those who were least active.

There is some evidence that physical activity is associated with a reduced risk of lung cancer. In a 2016 meta-analysis of 25 observational studies, physical activity was associated with reduced risk of lung cancer among former and current smokers but was not associated with risk of lung cancer among non-smokers.

For several other cancers, there is more limited evidence of an association. These include certain cancers of the blood, as well as cancers of the pancreas, prostate, ovaries, thyroid, liver, and rectum.

What kind of exercise do I do?

Over the years I have done different kinds of exercise, yoga, and meditation. Over the last few years, I have been walking for 40–60 minutes seven days a week with my dogs. In addition, I do some intermittent higher-intensity exercise, but I have not been very regular at it. For some time, I had hired a trainer to teach me exercises twice a week. I do hot yoga four to five days a week in a studio. Before I go for any pilgrimage involving climbing mountains or a lot of walking (like Vaishno Devi temple, Tirupati Venkateshwara temple, Sabarimala Ayyappa temple, Kunjaragiri Durgaparameshwari temple near Udupi, Ramana Ashram in Tiruvannamalai), I prepare myself for about three months by running on a treadmill, jogging, and some weight lifting. In addition, I have been learning and practicing yoga and meditation in different ways since my high school days. I initially learned to do sun salutation (Surya Namaskar) in my physical education classes from Shri K S Rao at Pompeii High School, Talipady, India. Later, I learned yoga and meditation during medical school from Dr. Krishna Bhat, Ph.D. for about two years. I also learned meditation informally from my psychiatry professor, Dr. Sripathi Bhat in Manipal. Over the last two decades, I have been fortunate to learn yoga and meditation from three legends, Swami Ramdev, Sri Sri Ravishankar, and Sadhguru Jaggi Vasudev. In addition, I have learned the meaning, philosophy, and science of yoga aphorisms (*Yoga Sutras* by Sage Patanjali) from Sriram Sarvotham, Ph.D., and Swami Bodhananda.

Yoga Sutras by Sage Patanjali is universally considered the foundational text on yoga. It describes an eight-limbed system, the third of which is the discipline of yoga postures called asanas. This is some kind of mild exercise and stretching. My current routine is 30 minutes of yoga and meditation taught by Sadhguru with some elements of Sudarshan Kriya, walking for

40–60 minutes seven days a week, and exercise training two days a week, for one hour each time. Having two dogs gives me additional reasons to walk. My dogs, Sophie and Charlie, add to my joy of walking. It is no surprise that my mentor, Dr. Oreopoulos, told me once, 'You don't know what love means till you own a dog'. It is important to do these activities every day, seven days a week, at the same time.

vii. Sleep for healing and prevention of cancer: *Good sleep, both in terms of time and quality, might help you heal. Sleep around seven hours a day*

Sleep is the most indispensable part of human life. We spend almost one-third of our life sleeping. We restore and recharge ourselves after a good sleep. It is believed that not sleeping well for long can cause many diseases. Published literature on the relationship between sleep duration and cancer risk is unclear. A meta-analysis published in 2018 by Chen and colleagues in BMC Cancer journal did not show any relation to sleep duration. There are theories of sleep habits, the release of melatonin, levels of sex hormones in the body, and cancer risk. However, there is no clear literature to make conclusive suggestions. But it stands to logic that good sleep is good for the body and sleep deprivation cannot be good.

For cancer patients, sometimes it is difficult to sleep well easily. The therapies sometimes disrupt your sleep-wake pattern. If you become sleep-deprived, you might end up feeling more tired, and coping with cancer becomes more difficult. Some patients sleep more than usual to repair their bodies.

I used to sleep seven to eight hours during my treatment, and after that, I had a good sleep pattern, which helped me to fight the illness and get treatment. When I could not sleep, I would listen to or recite chants, spiritual songs, or soft music, which would ensure infinite power within me and help me slip into sleep. My colleague, Late Dr. Brinker, had warned me not to watch TV if I could not get sleep. Often, I would read the second chapter of the Bhagavad Gita if I had a problem falling asleep. I would read a random page of the book, and I used to feel that I had found the answer to my problems. I would read till I felt sleepy again. I would recommend you read a scripture of your choice or any of your favorite books.

A few techniques for sleeping include inhaling a deep breath in and exhaling a deep breath out to calm your mind and eliminate excessive thoughts. When you are in bed, prepare for sleep by taking about 11 long deep breaths in and exhaling out, keeping your awareness of your breath. The inhalation is the universal force increasing your strength inside, and the exhalation is taking your toxins away. You can practice this anytime and feel relaxed and energized.

Another technique is to visualize yourself sleeping in the lap of your beloved one, the Divine, or your Guru, taking a few long breaths in and out while sleeping. You will quickly fall asleep. Just before sleeping, do something that uplifts your consciousness, like listening to spiritual discourses, music, spiritual songs, or just a few rounds of conscious breathing.

Some practice affirmations before going to bed. Some write down three to ten things they are grateful for before going to bed. Some write down three things that went well that day. There are times I have done some relaxation techniques soon after going to bed. One of the relaxation techniques that I initially learned from my psychiatry professor in medical school was to tighten my feet, ankles, legs, knees, thighs, hips, back, stomach, chest, shoulders, fingers, hands, arms, shoulders, back of the neck, front of the neck, back of the head, the face, and the scalp in that order and then to relax in the opposite order to relax the whole body. I have heard this relaxation technique from others as well since then. I have done this and taught this to others. I have found it helpful. Try it on yourself and see if you like it. Do it yourself or have someone with expertise teach you. One of the doctors with expertise in cancer prevention had recommended melatonin for sleep and also for cancer prevention. This doctor had a very holistic approach to cancer prevention. It comes in different strengths and is available over the counter. I randomly take melatonin whenever I feel like it. I take 10 mg tablets, probably three to four times a month. You can take in whatever dose pleases you or works for you. You don't have to take it if you don't want to take it. But it is important to sleep well to feel rested adequately. A rested body is a healing body, and a rested mind is a happy mind.

Chapter Nine

Cancer Screening for Prevention and Early Diagnosis

Cancer screening guidelines from US Preventive Services Task Force (USPSTF):

T his section has been reproduced from the USPSTF website. USP-STF allows authors to reproduce it without editing it. I could have just asked you to go to their website, but I thought I would make it easier for you by reproducing it since they allow it.

https://www.uspreventiveservicestaskforce.org/uspstf/recommendation/cervical-cancer-screening

Once a person gets one cancer, in addition to surveillance for recurrence of that cancer, we should also be vigilant in screening for other cancers. The U.S. Preventive Services Task Force (USPSTF) is an independent, volunteer panel of national experts in prevention and evidence-based medicine. Based on the level of evidence of benefit of a test, the USPSTF assigns one of five letter grades (A, B, C, D, or I).

USPTSF recommends to offer or provide grade A and B service.

For services graded C, USPSTF recommends offering or providing this service for selected patients depending on individual circumstances.

The USPSTF recommends against the service graded D since there is moderate or high certainty that the service has no net benefit or that the harms outweigh the benefits.

The USPSTF concludes that the current evidence is insufficient to assess the balance of benefits and harms of the service graded I. Evidence is lacking of poor quality, or conflicting, and the balance of benefits and harms cannot be determined. If grade I service is offered, patients should understand the uncertainty about balancing benefits and harms.

Recommendation Summary

Cervical Cancer (2018):

Women aged 21 to 65 years: The USPSTF recommends screening for cervical cancer every 3 years with cervical cytology alone in women aged 21 to 29 years. For women aged 30 to 65 years, the USPSTF recommends screening every 3 years with cervical cytology alone, every 5 years with high-risk human papillomavirus (hrHPV) testing alone, or every 5 years with hrHPV testing in combination with cytology (co-testing). See the Clinical Considerations section for the relative benefits and harms of alternative screening strategies for women 21 years or older. (Grade A)

Women younger than 21 years: The USPSTF recommends against screening for cervical cancer in women younger than 21 years. (Grade D)

Women who have had a hysterectomy: The USPSTF recommends against screening for cervical cancer in women who have had a hysterectomy with removal of the cervix and do not have a history of a high-grade precancerous lesion (i.e., cervical intraepithelial neoplasia [CIN] grade 2 or 3) or cervical cancer. (Grade D)

Women older than 65 years: The USPSTF recommends against screening for cervical cancer in women older than 65 years who have had adequate prior screening and are not otherwise at high risk for cervical cancer. See the Clinical Considerations section for discussion of adequate prior screening and risk factors that support screening after age 65 years. (Grade D)

Pancreatic Cancer (2019):

The USPSTF recommends against screening for pancreatic cancer in asymptomatic adults (Grade D).

Prostate Cancer: Screening (2018)

Men aged 55 to 69 years: For men aged 55 to 69 years, the decision to undergo periodic prostate-specific antigen (PSA)-based screening for prostate cancer should be an individual one. Before deciding whether to be screened, men should have an opportunity to discuss the potential benefits and harms of screening with their clinician and to incorporate their values and preferences in the decision. Screening offers a small potential benefit of reducing the chance of death from prostate cancer in some men. However, many men will experience potential harms of screening, including false-positive results that require additional testing and possible prostate biopsy; overdiagnosis and overtreatment; and treatment complications, such as incontinence and erectile dysfunction. In determining whether this service is appropriate in individual cases, patients and clinicians should consider the balance of benefits and harms on the basis of family history, race/ethnicity, comorbid medical conditions, patient values about the benefits and harms of screening and treatment-specific outcomes, and other health needs. Clinicians should not screen men who do not express a preference for screening. (Grade C)

Men 70 years and older: The USPSTF recommends against PSA-based screening for prostate cancer in men 70 years and older. (Grade D)

Skin Cancer Prevention: Behavioral Counseling (2018)

Young adults, adolescents, children, and parents of young children: The USPSTF recommends counseling young adults, adolescents, children, and parents of young children about minimizing exposure to ultraviolet (UV) radiation for persons aged 6 months to 24 years with fair skin types to reduce their risk of skin cancer. (Grade B).

Adults older than 24 years with fair skin types: The USPSTF recommends that clinicians selectively offer counseling to adults older than 24 years with fair skin types about minimizing their exposure to UV radiation to reduce risk of skin cancer. Existing evidence indicates that the net benefit of counseling all adults older than 24 years is small. In determining whether counseling is appropriate in individual cases, patients and clinicians should consider the presence of risk factors for skin cancer. See the Clinical Considerations section for information on risk assessment. (Grade C).

Adults:

The USPSTF concludes that the current evidence is insufficient to assess the balance of benefits and harms of counseling adults about skin self-examination to prevent skin cancer. (Grade I). See the Clinical Considerations section for suggestions for practice regarding the I statement.

Risk Assessment: Ultraviolet radiation exposure during childhood and adolescence increases risk of skin cancer later in life, especially when more severe damage occurs. Persons with fair skin type (light hair and eye color, freckles, those who sunburn easily) are at increased risk of skin cancer. Persons who use tanning beds and those with a history of sunburns or previous skin cancer are also at greatly increased risk of skin cancer. Other factors that increase risk include an increased number of nevi (moles) and atypical nevi, family history of skin cancer, HIV infection, and history of receiving an organ transplant.

Behavioral Counseling: Behavioral counseling interventions target sun protection behaviors to reduce UV radiation exposure, including use of broad-spectrum sunscreen with a sun-protection factor of 15 or greater; wearing hats, sunglasses, or sun-protective clothing; avoiding sun exposure; seeking shade during midday hours (10 am to 4 pm); and avoiding indoor tanning use.

Ovarian Cancer: Screening (2018)

Asymptomatic women: The USPSTF recommends against screening for ovarian cancer in asymptomatic women. This recommendation applies to asymptomatic women who are not known to have a high-risk hereditary cancer syndrome. (Grade D)

Thyroid Cancer: Screening (2018)

Adults: The USPSTF recommends against screening for thyroid cancer in asymptomatic adults. (Grade D)

Skin Cancer: Screening (2023)

Asymptomatic adults: The USPSTF concludes that the current evidence is insufficient to assess the balance of benefits and harms of visual skin examination by a clinician to screen for skin cancer in adults. (Grade I)

Colorectal Cancer: Screening (2016)

This topic is being updated.

Adults aged 50 to 75 years: The USPSTF recommends screening for colorectal cancer starting at age 50 years and continuing until age 75 years. The risks and benefits of different screening methods vary. See the Clinical Considerations section and the Table for details about screening strategies. (Grade A).

Adults aged 76 to 85 years: The decision to screen for colorectal cancer in adults aged 76 to 85 years should be an individual one, taking into account the patient's overall health and prior screening history. Adults in this age group who have never been screened for colorectal cancer are more likely to benefit. Screening would be most appropriate among adults who 1) are healthy enough to undergo treatment if colorectal cancer is detected and 2) do not have comorbid conditions that would significantly limit their life expectancy. (Grade C).

Aspirin Use to Prevent Cardiovascular Disease and Colorectal Cancer: Preventive Medication (2016)

Adults aged 50 to 59 years with a ≥10% 10-year cardiovascular disease risk: The USPSTF recommends initiating low-dose aspirin use for the primary prevention of cardiovascular disease (CVD) and colorectal cancer (CRC) in adults aged 50 to 59 years who have a 10% or greater 10-year CVD risk, are not at increased risk for bleeding, have a life expectancy of at least 10 years, and are willing to take low-dose aspirin daily for at least 10 years. (Grade B)

Adults aged 60 to 69 years with a ≥10% 10-year CVD risk: The decision to initiate low-dose aspirin use for the primary prevention of CVD and CRC in adults aged 60 to 69 years who have a 10% or greater 10-year CVD risk should be an individual one. Persons who are not at increased risk for bleeding, have a life expectancy of at least 10 years, and are willing to take low-dose aspirin daily for at least 10 years are more likely to benefit. Persons who place a higher value on the potential benefits than the potential harms may choose to initiate low-dose aspirin. (Grade C).

Adults aged 70 years or older: The current evidence is insufficient to assess the balance of benefits and harms of initiating aspirin use for the primary prevention of CVD and CRC in adults aged 70 years or older. (Grade I).

Adults younger than 50 years: The current evidence is insufficient to assess the balance of benefits and harms of initiating aspirin use for the primary prevention of CVD and CRC in adults younger than 50 years. (Grade I).

Breast Cancer: Screening

Women aged 50 to 74 years: The USPSTF recommends biennial screening mammography for women aged 50 to 74 years. (Grade B).

Women aged 40 to 49 years: The decision to start screening mammography in women prior to age 50 years should be an individual one. Women who place a higher value on the potential benefit than the potential harms may choose to begin biennial screening between the ages of 40 and 49 years. • For women who are at average risk for breast cancer, most of the benefit of mammography results from biennial screening during ages 50 to 74 years. Of all of the age groups, women aged 60 to 69 years are most likely to avoid breast cancer death through mammography screening. While screening mammography in women aged 40 to 49 years may reduce the risk for breast cancer death, the number of deaths averted is smaller than that in older women and the number of false-positive results and unnecessary biopsies is larger. The balance of benefits and harms is likely to improve as women move from their early to late 40s. • In addition to false-positive results and unnecessary biopsies, all women undergoing regular screening mammography are at risk for the diagnosis and treatment of noninvasive and invasive breast cancer that would otherwise not have become a threat to their health, or even apparent, during their lifetime (known as "overdiagnosis"). Beginning mammography screening at a younger age and screening more frequently may increase the risk for overdiagnosis and subsequent overtreatment. • Women with a parent, sibling, or child with breast cancer are at higher risk for breast cancer and thus may benefit more than average-risk women from beginning screening in their 40s. Go to the Clinical Considerations section for information on implementation of the C recommendation. (Grade C).

All women: The USPSTF concludes that the current evidence is insufficient to assess the benefits and harms of digital breast tomosynthesis (DBT) as a primary screening method for breast cancer. (Grade I).

Women with dense breasts: The USPSTF concludes that the current evidence is insufficient to assess the balance of benefits and harms of adjunctive screening for breast cancer using breast ultrasonography, magnetic resonance imaging, DBT, or other methods in women identified to have dense breasts on an otherwise negative screening mammogram. (Grade I)

Women aged 75 years or older: The USPSTF concludes that the current evidence is insufficient to assess the balance of benefits and harms of screening mammography in women aged 75 years or older. (Grade I)

Lung Cancer: Screening (2013)

Adults Aged 55-80, with a History of Smoking: The USPSTF recommends annual screening for lung cancer with low-dose computed tomography (LDCT) in adults aged 55 to 80 years who have a 30 pack-year smoking history and currently smoke or have quit within the past 15 years. Screening should be discontinued once a person has not smoked for 15 years or develops a health problem that substantially limits life expectancy or the ability or willingness to have curative lung surgery. (Grade B).

Oral Cancer: Screening (2013)

Asymptomatic Adults: The USPSTF concludes that the current evidence is insufficient to assess the balance of benefits and harms of screening for oral cancer in asymptomatic adults. (Grade I).

Readers are encouraged to go to for current recommendations since recommendations change sometimes as new scientific evidence becomes available. Other organizations also have screening guidelines that are available online.

Chapter Ten

Summary of Cancer Prevention

Cancer prevention interventions:
Important interventions fall under these categories.

Avoid smoking: Smoking in associated with higher risk of lung cancer, mouth cancer, throat cancer, esophageal and stomach cancer, colon cancer, kidney cancer, urinary bladder cancer, cancer of the uterus, ovarian cancer and certain leukemias. E-Cigarettes are also associated with higher cancer risk, though less than regular cigarettes. E-Cigarettes are associated with other additional risks associated with very high nicotine content, heavy metals and other toxic agents.

Avoid infections by vaccination. Human papilloma virus vaccine prevents cervical cancer and hepatitis B vaccine prevents liver cancers.

Avoid infections such as HIV, Hepatitis C and Hepatitis B by avoiding high risk sexual habits and intravenous drug abuse: AIDS (HIV) is associated with high risk of several malignancies and hence these malignancies are preventable by preventing acquiring these infection. Hepatitis C is also treatable and both hepatitis C and B are associated with liver cancer and are preventable.

Cancer Screening: Appropriate screening such as screening colonoscopy for screening or COLOGARD testing of the stools for colon cancer screening, mammogram for breast cancer screening, low dose lung

CT scan among smokers for lung cancer screening, PAP smear for cervical cancer screening and PSA blood test prostate cancer screening are some of the examples of tests to prevent cancers or for detection of pre-cancerous lesions or early cancers.

Surgeries: Prophylactic mastectomy of the opposite breast after having breast cancer on one side is common these days. Rarely people chose to have bilateral prophylactic mastectomy if they are at high risk for developing one.

Anticancer lifestyle changes for cancer prevention: Cancer prevention involves harmonizing the five elements of the body with those of the universe. When there is harmony among these five elements in the microcosm and macrocosm, there will be wellness and no cancer. When there is disharmony, there will be illness such as cancer. American Institute of Cancer Research has published ten recommendations for cancer prevention. Cancer prevention measures can also be described as those harmonizing the five elements, incorporating AICR guidelines and the pillars of Lifestyle medicine.

- Nutrition/Earth: Healthy, plant dominant diet with 7-10 servings of fruits and vegetables/day, eat whole grains and beans; limit red meat, processed food and fast foods; do not use nutritional supplements to prevent cancer.

- Nutrition/Water: Adequate intake of water and smoothies (~60 oz/day); avoid alcohol, sodas, sugary drinks, sweeteners and colors; limit juices; breast feeding.

- Smoke/Air: Breathing fresh air, avoid smoking and polluted air.

- Stress/Fire: Yoga, meditation, exercise, singing, chanting, dancing, laughing or some similar interventions to reduce stress and enhance a blissful life experience regularly.

- Space: The good company of and connection with friends and family; divine experience with prayer, chanting, self-study, self-inquiry, and meditation. This section will be discussed at greater depth later in the book under the section on 'Experiencing Infinity'.

- Appropriate cancer screening to detect precancerous lesions and early cancers so they can be dealt with before developing clinically manifest cancer.

I have put all these in a 00077777000 acronym to make it easier to remember

Dr Shetty's 00077777000 Program for Wellness

- 0 sodas and drinks with sugar or sweeteners
- 0 alcohol
- 0 smoking
- 7 servings of vegetables and fruits per day: Smoothie, and use your kitchen, keep it simple, positive nutritional excellence
- 7 hours or more of exercise/walking per week: Own a dog
- 7 hours or more of yoga/meditation/recreational reading/singing/dancing/laughing/prayer per week
- 7 hours or more of sleep per day: Go to bed early
- 7 hours or more of screen free time per week: Keep the phone aside
- 7000 steps a day: Walk daily at the same time, add steps at work

Be unconditionally happy like a baby

00077777000 Program for Wellness

SECTION 4:
A COMMONER'S EXPERIENCE OF INFINITY

Chapter Eleven

Definition of Infinity and GOD

He who choses 'The Infinite' has been chosen by 'The Infinite'

Sri Aurobindo

'Infinity' is the word I chose to describe that 'entity' or 'power' or 'spirit' within us and outside us all over the universe. The various synonyms of 'Infinity' are 'Brahman,' 'Supreme Lord,' 'Supreme God,' 'God,' and 'One.' Eckert Tolle calls it 'NOW'. Sikhs call it 'Ik' (which means 'one') or 'Ik Onkar'. Hindus, Jains, Sikhs, Buddhists, and others call it 'OM'. *Rig Veda*, one of the ancient sacred Hindu scriptures, states, 'The Supreme is One, sages/people call it different ways.' Christians may call 'him' as 'Jehovah', Muslims call it/him 'Allah', Jews, Baha'is, and people of other faiths call 'him' in their own ways. Many Hindus call 'it' with different names, some of them being Krishna, Krishna consciousness, Rama, Vishnu, Shiva, Brahma, Durga, Mother, Amma, Hanuman, Murugan, Ganapati, Surya, etc. Some disagree with those who worship God/Infinity in form and names. But according to one of the sacred Hindu scriptures, *Tulsi Ramayana*, it is a privilege to be able to see and sing about the attributeless God in form and name. Some see it as a necessity to experience God with attributes to access God. You need to have a glass if you want to offer someone water. You cannot provide water to your friend or guest without a glass or a bottle. (This example was given to Swami Chinmayananda by his Guru, Swami Tapovan Maharaj and the story's details are available online). It is a common practice among Hindus to worship God with attributes. Invoking the form of Jesus Christ and Mother Mary is a common practice among Christians by having the respective 'idols' in the forms of sculptures and paintings in churches and small personal idols or 'cross' in pendants and photos. Buddhists keep Buddha's idols in their houses and monasteries. Many see Infinity in prophets. Sometimes 'Infinity' comes into our lives as mother, father, guru, and friend. 'Infinity' might show up as food, water, air, shelter, or a 'divine voice' from somebody known or unknown. In the movie '*Life of Pi*', the main actor playing 'Pi Patel' expresses gratitude to God Vishnu for appearing as 'fish' when he had nothing else to eat in the middle of the ocean after the shipwreck. In Hindu scriptures, God Vishnu had once incarnated as a divine 'Fish (*Matsya*)'. Some of the secular words to indicate 'Infinity' are 'pure consciousness', 'witness consciousness', 'the truth', and 'awareness'. The experience of 'Infinity' is also described as 'truth-consciousness-bliss' ('*Sat-chit-ananda*').

Here is a peace chant on 'Infinity' [from Kenopanishad and Chandogya Upanishad (#2 in the glossary)]:

May my limbs, speech, life-force (Prana), sight, hearing, strength, and all my senses, gain in vigor. All is the Brahman (Supreme Lord, Infinity) of the Upanishads. May I never deny the Brahman/Infinity. May the Brahman/Infinity never deny me. May there be no denial of the Brahman/Infinity. May there be no separation from the Brahman/Infinity. May all the virtues manifest in me, who am devoted to the Atman (Higher Self). May thy manifest in me.

OM! PEACE! PEACE! PEACE!

This chant ends with the prayer for protection from three-fold miseries affecting the human body and mind, miseries affecting other living beings, and miseries such as natural calamities like earthquakes, floods, wildfires, tsunamis, etc.

What is Infinity/God?

'Ye, Children of Immortal Bliss' —Swami Vivekananda

'God' is well described in Kenopanishad (or Kena Upanishad), one of the Hindu scriptures, and in many other places. Kena in Sanskrit means 'by what', referring to the various things that we experience happen. A very brief description of this is that this is the command behind what makes the mind think, life force (Prana) move, eyes see, 'speech' speak, ears hear. That 'thing' is referred to as 'Brahman/Infinity'. I am calling it 'Infinity' in this book. Others have done it too.

'Infinity' is also described as OM. Transliteration of the most sacred mantra (also called root mantra), 'Ik Onkar', chanted by the Sikhs is 'true name, without fear and enmity (all-compassionate), one which transcends time, birth and death, self-existent, true today, true eternally and realized by Guru's grace.'

'Infinity' is also described as the 'Fourth (turiya) state', one beyond the wake, dream, and sleep states of the self. It is an experience of consciousness that is neither inwards, nor outwards, nor both. It is beyond cognition and beyond the absence of cognition. The senses cannot sense it, it is not known by comparison, deductive reasoning, or inference; it is indescribable, incomprehensible, and unthinkable. It is pure consciousness, the pure self that witnesses the self in the waking, dream, and sleep states. It is serene, tranquil, blissful. It is the ONE, one without a second. It makes us realize that material life is an illusion and temporary. This is the real or true Self that is to be realized. It is also described as AUM, followed by silence. 'A' represents the waking state of the self, 'U' represents the dream state of the self, 'M' represents the sleep state of the self and silence represents the pure, infinite truth of the unmanifest self that witnesses the self, manifesting in the waking, dream, and sleep states. (Ref: Mandukya Upanishad in verse 7 and Ashtavakra Gita 1:12). OM is described in a lot of other scriptures. Sadhguru claims that Om (Aum) has found its way in the more recent Abrahamic faiths as well. Many yoga practitioners chant Om and hence OM is easily the universal message of peace to be united with the universal ONE and has transcended all faiths. More curious readers are recommended to read the book, "Enlightenment without GOD" (ISBN 13: 978-089389-084-1).

A more precise definition of God is...

'The all consummate definition (Ref: *Taittiriya Upanishad 2.1.1*) **of 'God/Ishwara/Brahman/Infinity is Truth, Knowledge, and Infinite'** (*Satyam, Jnanam, Anantam Brahma*) and it is experienced as 'truth, cosmic intelligence, and bliss' (*Sat, Chit, Ananda*). *Satyam*, is the eternal, unchanging truth that exists. Body and mind change every day and hence are not the eternal truths. *Jnanam* means 'knowledge', referring to the knowledge of pure consciousness in which my body is situated, in this context. *Anantam* means 'one without a limit', referring to 'unlimited in space, time, and object'. 'Unlimited in space' means Brahman is all-pervading, omnipresent, not just 'up there', not just in heaven, but everywhere including here. 'Unlimited in time' means Brahman is eternal without a beginning or end, Brahman is available to experience now, today, tomorrow, and every day in this life, not just after death. 'Unlimited in object' means that Brahman is beyond the definition of an object. Wave is nothing but water, there is no 'second thing' other than water. Brahman is 'ALL', ONE without a second, non-dual.

For ease of understanding to the secular readers, I described Brahman or God as 'Infinity', knowing that 'Infinity' does not describe it all. 'Infinity' is not my discovery or invention; others use this term as well. For the secular people, Brahman is the Godless 'Infinity'.

Chapter Twelve

Different Methods for Liberation From Cancer and Experiencing INFINITY

- Path of love (devotion) towards God: Prayer and devotion to God to experience Infinity

- Path of action (karma): Performing day to day activities with gratitude as an offering to God to experience Infinity

- Path of contemplation: Unconditional happiness and unconditional love to experience Infinity

- Path of knowledge: Healing with non-duality to experience Infinity

    ○ Six verses leading to Infinity

    ○ Who am I?: Self-inquiry to experience Infinity

- Buddhist approach to experience Infinity: I am the 'awakened (Buddha)'

- Yoga and meditation to experience Infinity

- Ik Onkar/AUM/OM to experience Infinity

- Universal ways to dissolve into Infinity

Like we all know, all rivers lead to the same ocean, the same pool of water. All religions of the world lead to the same ONE God. Paths are many, but the destination is the same. Broadly speaking, there are three types of religious practices. The most common practice is the practice of devotion. This is a very well-organized, conventional way of practicing religion and is practiced in Christianity, Islam, Judaism, a large majority of Hindus practicing dualism and also others, Sikhs, Jains, and others. The only requirement for this practice is the 'faith' in God. The strength of this method is that it is conventional and is heavily institutionalized. There are plenty of resources to support this in every religion, all over the world. My only request is to be all-inclusive and know that all faiths and practices lead to the same God. No path is better than the other. There cannot be a different God for each religion. People pray differently, some pray to God to solve their problems, some repeat God's names and feel the 'Infinity', some sing on God and experience 'Infinity', some think of God every minute they are awake and experience 'Infinity'. Sant Kabir Das, an Indian mystic and poet of the 15th century CE, said, "When I walk, I think I am circumambulating the Lord; when I work, I think I am serving God; and when I sleep, I think I am offering Him my obeisances. In this manner, I perform no activity other than that which is offered to Him."

The next practice is an experience-based practice like Buddhism and Yoga and some philosophies of Hinduism. This is experiential and hence cannot be questioned except by those who do not experience it. Not everybody can experience it. This is also practiced by millions of people all over the world, some see it as spiritual and not religious.

The third practice is 'knowledge based' or 'self-based' and is available in this life and in this world. This practice requires knowledge of the self, the knowledge that the real truth of 'I' is infinitely divine. This is practiced by the non-dualists and mainly by non-dualistic Hindus, Buddhists, and Sikhs. There is some element of non-dualism in Sufism, Christianity, and Judaism as well even though they are mainly dualistic faiths. This is not experience-based and hence is accessible to everyone without the prerequisite of faith in God. I have discussed this in many ways in the entire book and hence will not dwell on it here. These methods are not mutually exclusive and most people practice all three methods at different times in their lives usually focussing on one method more than others.

A common doubt is "Is the experience of 'Infinity' possible for a commoner like you and me?" I do not know the revealed scriptures, I am not a saint, I am not an enlightened person, I do not know the Sanskrit language, I do not have superpowers. I have read that such enlightened experiences are experienced by rare people. Most of us are not one of those. I certainly am not. Simply put, do I have access to God? My challenge to you is that we all have access to God in this life, right now, right here. The 'path of knowledge' is a way for the commoners to experience 'Infinite God' in this life and be benefitted from it. In other words, we are talking about democratizing God in this life.

Experiencing Infinity by divinizing our day-to-day activities:

I have initially written on simpler methods of experiencing Infinity by following one of these four pathways (love, action, meditation, and knowledge) and divinizing them:

1. Divinizing our love towards God by devotion and prayers,

2. Divinizing our action by practicing gratitude and doing day to day activities as a service to God,

3. Divinizing contemplation and meditation by practicing 'unconditional infinite happiness and love', and

4. Divinizing knowledge of the 'self' by knowing about healing from non-duality by knowing that the self is 'Infinity'.

These experiences are available to commoners like most of us because we already do these. We just have to look at them from a divine angle. These are ways to experience Infinity 24/7.

Profound ways of experiencing Infinity:

A little bit more profound ways of experiencing 'Infinity' are by following the paths of self-experience and acquiring knowledge that the 'Self is Divine.' Some of these methods include knowing the methods of self-inquiry and yoga from the eastern Hindu wisdom. I also brought in 'I am the Awakened (Buddha)' from Buddhist philosophy. These are more profound concepts that need to be read, studied, and contemplated slowly. This is not a quick read like a novel if you want to personally experience it.

Some ways of experiencing Infinity for common people, like you and I are described in the following categories:

a. Path of love towards God: prayer and devotion to God to experience Infinity

Prayers are really powerful. I have deliberately repeated this section on prevention and experiencing Infinity because it does both. I pray every day. Different people pray differently. Some pray for themselves and don't believe in others praying for them. Many believe in their own prayers and also derive strength in others praying for them. Lots of shrines have a system of praying for people to get better. And some simply don't believe in prayers, they just believe in actions (karma path to realizing God). Some others believe in praying to God, surrendering to God, and asking God to heal. They get the strength to heal from total surrender to God. Such people 'beg' God either for themselves or others. These are mainly 'dualists' who see God and themselves separate from each other and pray to God for favors. There are 'dualists' in almost every faith in the world. It is the fundamental response from every person who believes in God as their ultimate savior.

I know that many have prayed for me. I know many of my patients, patients' friends, my friends, and friends' friends have prayed in some Churches in Dallas. Thanks to all of them, I have not had a chance to thank them personally. Some believe in prayers, meditations, chants, and the study of scriptures to unveil the soul, God, infinite energy within them. Such people may not ask God to make them better, they may at best pray for strength.

Many people just meditate upon and invoke the 'eternal strength' within them. I believe that the belief in non-duality is very strong; those people will only invoke the 'strength' within them without begging God to heal them. Such people should not be worried. Worrying about the outcome would be questioning their very belief. Finally, some people just believe they have the infinite strength to heal and do all the right things to get better. Among these different approaches is one better than the other? I do not know. Whatever works for you is fine. Whatever you feel comfortable with is fine. Whatever gives you strength is the right approach. There is nothing much to choose between the 'dualistic approach' and 'non-dualistic approach'. I feel I benefited from both approaches. I like to believe that I am a non-dualist. But I also know that I go back and forth between being a dualist and non-dualist. Even the saints professing non-dualism like Adi Shankara and others have been the greatest devotees practicing dualism in some ways.

The Hindu philosophy recommends one or all of the different paths to experience God. Those different paths are paths of devotion (bidirectional love towards God, *bhakti*), work (*karma*), contemplation (*Raja yoga*), and path of knowledge (*jnana*). Any one or all the paths are fine depending upon your strengths, weaknesses, comfort level, and experience. But there is a reference to the greatest of the geniuses (Jnanis) eventually becoming devotees of God in every era of mankind. Some of these examples are Adi Shankara in the current era who surrendered to God with features and names like Vishnu, Shiva, and Devi after writing extensively on attribute-less God and non-dualistic philosophy, Saint Shukha who became Lord Krishna's devotee after being the greatest genius, King Janaka who worshipped Lord Rama, and Sanat Kumara and his associates who became great devotees of God despite establishing themselves as the greatest geniuses of their respective eras. There is a lot written about worshipping God with a name and repeating the name of God in your favorite way. People refer to God by different names such as Krishna, Rama, Vishnu, Shiva, Devi, Hanuman, Brahman, and many others if you are a Hindu. Christians may refer to God as Jesus Christ, Mother Mary, or Jehovah. Muslims may refer to God as Allah. Jews, Jains, Buddhists, Sikhs, Bahais, native Indians of the US and Canada, Mayans and Aztecs of Central America and Mexico, Samoans, Incans, Polynesians, and all the different people of the world have their own unique ways of worshipping and addressing God in their own way. Lots of people of all faiths simply refer to God as the 'Man up there'. In other words, even the faiths professing worshipping God without attributes refer to God as 'Man up there'. Knowingly or unknowingly, everyone goes back and forth between worshipping God with form and without attributes. Hindus do not just refer to God as the 'Man up there', but they get the credit for worshipping God with women's name and form, man's name and form, animal's name and form, and without attributes. Hindus refer to God as a baby and also as a lover with divine love. Sometimes God comes to us as a parent, teacher, or friend. I have heard Swami Bodhananda say that God's name is always available to us to recite and repeat even if we may not know how to feel and see God ourselves. Hence many believe that repeating God's name is extremely powerful. If you study Swami Prabhupada, he taught people to repeat the Hare Krishna maha-mantra thousands of times till they experience ecstasy. Many people were able to quit hard drugs like cocaine, heroin, and 'ecstasy' by reciting this maha-mantra thousand of times every day because they were able to experience ecstasy without using 'Ecstasy'. That was the power of repeating God's names, that is the power of meditation.

At a personal level, I feel that I believe in the 'non-dualistic approach' and invoke God within me and leave the rest to God. I try not to beg God to make me better. I did not beg God to save me. But I did go through a lot of pain during chemotherapy and radiation before having surgery. I also went through a lot of pain after surgery. I tried hard to 'not experience the pain' by trying to separate my body from my 'Self' and trying to convince myself that I am the Atma/Self/soul and pain is in my body which is not the real me. I meditated, prayed, and invoked the God within me. The pain was nerve-wracking sometimes and I felt that I was not strong or evolved enough to separate 'me' from my physical body. During these hours I did become dualistic and begged God for strength. I begged God to take away my pain. I have caught myself begging for my mother, crying out aloud 'ammaaa...' when I was in pain.

If this means I did not believe in God within me, I feel that I did believe that there was a 'Big God' who was stronger than the God within me. I may have separated the water in the wave from the water in the ocean! I don't know. All I know is pain really hurts. 'Pain in the butt' is the real pain in the butt! It really hurts. I did not like the language that Lance Armstrong used in his book even though I do not doubt his true experience and feelings. Sometimes using colloquial words really conveys the point and that is what he did in his book and that is what I did here.

Back to the issue of whether prayers help, I believe they do. I believe that it helped me. Research has shown that support groups help improve the outcomes in those who participate in them. My suggestion is to personalize your way of praying. If you feel comfortable, allow or request others to pray for you. If you feel uncomfortable with strangers knowing about your personal life, ask for anonymous prayers. If you feel that prayer is strictly personal communion between you and God, discourage the mass prayers and pray alone in your privacy. Prayer does not have to be transactional. Exploring the possibilities in life is trying to experience God (Brahman). The physical body in me tries to survive from the risks of destruction of my body from the different dangers in this world. The physical body in me does everything to survive and wants to give the best possibility of the best outcome by getting the best treatment in the world in the best hospital in the world by the best doctors in the world. Physical being in me wants to play a team sport by building the best team in the world to give me the best chance of conquering cancer in me. When the physical being in me surrenders to the superpower guarding everything that I have, including my body and mind which includes cancer in my body, I don't have to worry about anything. The mental being in me acquires all the knowledge to do whatever it can be done to save me from cancer. But the spiritual being in me itself is the omnipotent, omniscient God (Brahman) and hence I do not have to worry about cancer or any worldly problems. The mental being in me knows that I am the reflection of infinite consciousness and is aware that I should be aligned in the correct angle to get the best reflection of God.

The spiritual being in me realizes that it is only my physical body that gets sick and has the risk of dying, the spiritual being in me is never scared of getting sick, never scared of cancer, never scared of pain, never scared of death. The spiritual being in me is aware that the real 'I' never gets sick, I never get cancer, I can never die and 'I' am 'Infinity'. Brahman in me is aware that I am the light of the lights, strongest among the strong, best among the doctors, of the water I am the mighty ocean, of the mountains I am the mighty Himalayas, of the medicines I'm the best medicine and of the God I am the supreme God. I am time, I am timeless, and I am the beginning, middle, and end, I am birthless, deathless and I'm fearless and I am the truth and the only truth. When I know this I have nothing to worry about because what I see and what I feel is limited, temporary, and finite and hence not the infinite truth. The real truth is the pure consciousness in me. Hence when I pray all I have to do is to surrender to God, offer my body and mind to God, and lose the boundary between myself and God.

God says in chapter 2 of the Gita, 'the real me cannot be cut, cannot be made wet, cannot be burned, it is eternal, it is all pervading'. We should do our duties not so much with passion, but with tranquility (equanimity of mind) as a service to God. If we do everything including eating, breathing, drinking, taking medicines as service to God, we would only do the right thing, we would only do the best thing in the world.

For those who are eager to help patients with prayers, please do so, but remember to give space to the patients. Please remember to respect a patient's faith, belief, and privacy. Please remember that in this world there are different ways of praying and different ways of worshipping. There are different names to the same almighty. There are different paths to the same destination. All the paths are valid. All the different rivers lead to the same mighty ocean. Please do not impose your way on anybody, neither the patient nor the family member nor your friend. Imposing your faith on a vulnerable person is equivalent to abuse, it is social injustice. Please remember that you are not helping anybody when you impose your faith on a patient or family member of a patient. If you want to help and if you believe that your prayer has value, please pray on your own. If you wish, you can tell the patient that you are praying for his/her health and recovery. There is no need to confuse and disrespect the patient and family by imposing your faith on them. Let them pray in their own way. Finally, please remember that it is not about you, it is about the patient. Your intentions may be good, but don't impose your help if it suffocates the patient.

Even though I used to pray, I used to feel grateful and awkward at the same time when people said that they would pray for me. But I know lots of people of different faiths have prayed for me and I am extremely grateful to them. I know people have prayed for me in many temples, churches, and houses in India, the United States, and probably elsewhere. I know that some people have cried for me. Some of these people are not even those who I have dealt with on a day-to-day basis, I may not even know some of them. Maybe that is why I am alive today! Like my father-in-law said, I had so much goodwill from so many people that it would not go to waste. It indeed didn't!

I liked having a spiritual Guru in Swami Sarveshananda of Chinmaya Mission Dallas, Fort Worth, who was extremely compassionate and helpful. He came to my home to bless me, guide me, clear some doubts for me and my family, and was always there for me! Thank you, Swamiji! My father-in-law once told me that God made a mistake in getting ready to 'take me to Him', and then 'spit me back' when he realized his mistake. It makes me feel special to be the 'saliva' of God. It makes me feel good knowing that I am part of God. It gives me infinite strength. My faith teaches the non-duality concept. This is an infinitely powerful concept when one is sick. If God is in me, why worry? When God is in me, I don't have to go pillar to post seeking God. I just have to unveil the God in me. When God is in me I already have infinite strength, I just have to unveil it, transcend into it and *be* it, *be the Infinity*.

I prayed to Goddess Durga and Lord Hanuman, both divine manifestations of 'Infinite strength (*Shakti*)', healing, and 'compassion'. I sang the devotional song *Hanuman Chalisa* every day for many months and I still sing it often since it makes me feel energized. I sing it when I am happy, I sing it when I feel vulnerable. I did beg God for strength to heal me and to tolerate pain. I did not pray to God to save my life since I felt that God knew better when and how I should die. My suggestion is to pray in your own way that empowers you and that makes you feel connected to the 'Infinite Divine Energy' irrespective of your faith. If you don't want to pray, you don't have to do it. If you feel like begging God to save you, beg God. There is no wrong way to pray. I know some get upset with God for allowing the illness to come and some start questioning the existence of God. But I feel that it is better to pray and surrender to God during such challenging times so you will have a 'go-to person' to share the burden! If you believed in God before falling sick, I would recommend that you continue to pray. Faith in God should not be conditional and should not be transactional. Know that God does not prevent death and God does not prevent many things from happening. But these are very personal choices that one should exercise depending upon their beliefs, experiences, and knowledge.

One thing that I am very certain of is that you don't fall sick because you belong to or do not belong to one faith, you don't fall sick because you did not pray. You can make your own choices!

Does prayer heal one from cancer? Does prayer prevent cancer? These are difficult questions. There may not be scientifically proven answers to these questions. There is evidence that patients who are part of support groups do better than those who are not. I firmly believe that prayers strengthen our immune system and help prevent and heal cancers. I firmly believe that prayers helped me deal with problems in my life better and I think it will help you too. I think that prayer will help you lead a happier life. If you remain angry with God, there is a good possibility that you will remain angry with everything in life. It is unlikely that you will not see any problems in your life. All of us do. 'As long as there is life, there will always be a struggle,' according to Mr. Harivansh Rai Bacchan, father of the Bollywood legend Amitabh Bacchan. I loved the movie, 'Eat Love and Pray'. I recommend that you eat, love, and pray. Finally, pray 24/7 as Sant Kabir Das taught. Pray in your own way that empowers you and that makes you feel connected to 'Infinite Divine Energy' irrespective of your faith.

Let me quote one universal prayer that is a healing, transformational and meditative prayer that I chant every day.

"Lead us from untruth to truth, lead us from darkness to light, lead us from mortality to immortality."

b. Path of action (karma): Performing day to day activities with gratitude as an offering to God to experience Infinity

Being grateful for what has been given to you attracts more happiness in life while complaining about what has been taken away brings more sorrow. Jesus said, "Those who have will be given more, those who have not will be taken whatever they have." Mr. Harivansh Rai Bacchan also said, 'It is good if things go your way, but it is better if it does not go your way because going according to God's wish cannot be bad'.

Throughout my journey, I have been grateful to the Infinity, my spiritual Gurus, people around me especially my family, friends, and relatives, unknown well-wishers, my team of doctors, nurses, and each and every one who was there with me during this journey. I would like to advise you all to appreciate whatever is around and be genuinely grateful for whatever blessing is showered on you.

Gratitude removes several toxic emotions like envy, resentment, frustration, and regret. It rewires your brain and makes you feel more energized and keeps you out of grumbling and getting into self-pity and negativity. A positive aura is a must to heal and you must keep yourself away from people scaring and talking negatively about your health condition. In such conditions, instead of getting disturbed by their remarks, just take this opportunity to educate them. You can educate your family and friends about what cancer patients like to hear and do not like to hear. Most people mean well and are willing to learn. This is one way of converting a negative experience into an educational opportunity.

My gratitude practice during the journey used to be something like what I have mentioned below. You can make it yours in your own way. An attitude and expression of gratitude can be as follows:

Oh God/Infinity/'One'/'Unity',

Thank you for your blessings since I know that I can count on them.

Thank you for the wisdom that I have and many don't.

Thank you for giving me eyesight that I have and many don't.

Thank you for the ability to hear and listen that I have and many don't.

Thank you for giving me functioning hands that I have and many don't.

Thank you for giving me the ability to talk and walk that I have and many don't.

Thank you for giving me a loving spouse that I have and many don't.

Thank you for giving me children that I have and many don't.

Thank you for having my mother alive till the age of 88 years.

Thank you for having my father till the age of 96 years.

Thank you for giving me loving and supportive siblings that I have and many don't.

Thank you for giving me a loving family that I have and many don't.

Thank you for giving me caring friends that I have and many don't.

Thank you for giving me food to eat that I have and many don't.

Thank you for giving me a place to live that I have and many don't.

Thank you for giving me peace in life that I have and many don't

Thank you for what I have.

I know that I don't have everything that I desire, but I have a lot of things that I desire. I also know that many don't have what I do.

Thank you for your blessings.

Thank you for your blessings.

Thank you for your blessings.

Like this, I would soak into gratefulness and bask in the abundance showered on me by Infinite power. By doing this, I experienced a bounty of power to fight against cancer. Practicing gratitude is a very powerful way to be happy in life, it is a great way to be appreciative of people around us and a very good way to be content with our health irrespective of our health. Another approach I have taken is being optimistic, looking forward to better days when things are not going well, and being appreciative of the good moments.

c. Path of contemplation: Unconditional happiness and unconditional love to experience Infinity

Kids are unconditionally happy and cry only if there is a reason. We, the grown-ups have to remind ourselves that we can be happy too without looking for a reason to be so. It takes some contemplation, practice and meditation to experience unconditional bliss. Happiness is a choice that you have to make. Don't depend on circumstances or people to be happy. Just choose to be happy. Happiness and bliss are your default state. Happiness does not have to be conditional. You don't have to do anything to be happy. You just have to choose to be happy no matter what goes on around you. If everything is going well, it is another reason to be happy. If things are not so well, be happy that it is going to get better. Be happy that it is not that bad. If you are rich, there is no reason to be unhappy. If you are not, be happy looking for better days. Be happy with what you have because many don't have what you have. If you are well, be happy. If you are unwell, be happy that you are going to be better or because you are not that unwell. In other words, I chose to be happy unconditionally. In 1989, when I was having simple hernia surgery, my colleague Dr. Arati Tavargeri Shahade, who is a famous diabetologist in Pune, India, gave me a greeting card, which said the famous quote which goes as 'if you get better it is a reason to be happy, but if you don't get better and die, you will still be happy having fun in heaven'. At that time I did not realize how profound the message was, in fact, I felt creepy. But now I really understand it better. Thank you, Arati! You were mature beyond your age at that time. I was not.

You still are! You impress me even today with your dedication to excellence and 'Infinity' in your field. I have heard cancer survivors say that it was the best thing that happened to them. I would not say that. It is terrible to have cancer. It is terrible to go through chemotherapy, radiation, and surgery. It is terrible to have pain. It is terrible to go through the uncertainty of life and death when you have a young wife and children. Of course, some good things come out of this unfamiliar situation. You learn to swim when you are thrown into the water. Some doctors say that they became better doctors after they went through a serious illness. I want to believe that I was already a compassionate and knowledgeable doctor. I don't say that I became a better doctor. I already used to manage pain as best as I could. But I now know better about how pain hurts from my own experience. I do know what pain in the 'behind' is.

One thing I have started doing is telling patients that 'I have first-hand experience of going through pain and that I have a feel for what they are going through'. I also have started coaching patients on how to deal with pain. There is hardly anything good about suffering and pain. It teaches some life lessons. It does make us realize the privileges that many times we take for granted. But there are easier ways to learn them. I know people who are taller, smarter, healthier, and wealthier than me. But I also know people who don't have what I am blessed with. I know people who drive better cars than me. But all cars have to follow the same speed limit, follow the same traffic rules, and share the same roads. At least for now, unless Elon Musk does something magical! I also know people who are unable to drive and want to drive. So why not be happy with whatever you have. Reading the book, '*My Life*' by President Clinton was an eye-opener. His biological father died before he was born. He had a stepfather who was abusive towards his wife and was an alcoholic. But apparently, he was very loving! So President Clinton took his stepfather's last name since he had never seen his biological father, Mr. Blythe! President Clinton said something very real. He said, 'if you look around you, you will realize that most people have some problem or the other that they have decided to live with, without complaining about it.'

There is a great sentence in Hindu scriptures, '*Tat Tvam Asi*'. That means, 'That thou art' which means, 'You Are That (divine reality)'. It means 'you are divine'. All of us have a divine soul, divine self, Atman. Our soul is a part of 'God'. I have interpreted this great sentence as 'There is divinity in everything and everybody', 'There is good in every person, everything and every situation'. I have learned to see the good things in life and be happy unconditionally. The expression, 'count your blessings' is another way of saying this. Counting your blessings is an extremely common tool for getting through adversity in the western world. The great sentence, 'That thou art', is extremely profound and empowering. Not only that it means 'you are that divine reality', it means that the real 'you' is divine. You are not your mind, body, or intellect, you are not what you feel with your eyes, nose, tongue, ear, and skin; you are not your mind, you are the pure consciousness, you are the divine self, you are the 'awareness', the pure self, the pure truth, the pure infinite truth, the infinite potential, the real you are the Brahman, the God, the Infinity. The real God is within us. The real God is you. *"All of 'you' is God"*. We don't have to wait for us to die and go to heaven to see God. The real God is right here, right now for you to feel and experience, right within you. In fact, your body is within the divine you. You are that truth, you are that knowledge that the 'real you' is the 'divine you'. You are that infinite self, one who is infinite in space, omnipresent; you are infinite in time. You are that infinite 'One', one without a second, one which is not separate from God, You are that, you are all. I can go on and on. But I am happy because I chose to be so.

You have the same choice that I have. Today, why don't you choose to be happy?

It is great to be happy, but it is important to have equanimity of mind. In the Bhagavad Gita, God told his disciple and friend: 'O Arjun, noblest amongst men, that person who is not affected by happiness and distress and remains steady in both, becomes eligible for liberation.'

God Krishna explains that both the sensations of happiness and distress are fleeting. In other words, both material happiness and distress are temporary. When we grow beyond what is ever-changing, we liberate ourselves from the material realities and experience the permanent bliss, our true nature. When we are in that state of bliss we get to the state of infinite bliss, eternal-sentient bliss (*sat-chit-ananda*). This state is our true nature. Hence, Swami Vivekananda addresses people by saying, "O ye children of immortal bliss." In layman's words, we learn to be in "unconditional happiness". When we learn to treat the opposites like heat and cold, wellness and illness, happiness and distress with equipoise, we will be "unconditionally happy". This is experiencing "Infinity". This is "eternal truth and permanent bliss".

"Above all the mantras I have given you, finally, I give you a mantra. No matter where you live and wherever you go, in any condition you are, even while you are crying, and you are crying in pain, agony, remember my words: Learn to be happy. No one makes you happy. No one has the power to insert happiness. There is no such pill, there is no such medicine that makes you happy. You have to learn to make yourself happy. So no matter where you go, learn to be happy. Happiness is a state of tranquility. It means don't allow anyone to disturb your mind."

This is from Swami Rama and is based on his lectures on Yoga Aphorisms by Sage Patanjali.

Do you know that the little kids are always happy? They don't need a reason to be happy. Happiness is their default state. They need a reason to be unhappy. If they cry, we look for a reason, such as wet diapers, belly pain (colic), or hunger! Otherwise, they are always happy, smiling, and playing. Now, see what happens when we grow older. We try to find ways to be happy! Does this mean that our default state changed from being happy to being unhappy? It looks like that happened at some time as we grew up without us knowing about it. This unhappiness in adult life, or 'needing some ways or means to be happy' in adults is due to the ignorance that crept into us. When we grow we want to be rich to be happy, we want a big house to be happy, we want a nice car to be happy, we want a pretty/handsome spouse to be happy, we want our children in famous schools to be happy, we want our children to be married to famous people to be happy, we want to have grandchildren to be happy, we want to take a vacation to be happy, we want a certain status to be happy, we want things to change to be happy! Isn't it strange that when the ever unchanging 'bliss' is in us 24/7, we keep going away, farther and farther to find ways to be happy? Bringing back this knowledge that our default state is true 'bliss' will solve the problem of unhappiness in this world. That will bring us joy without a condition. We would be unconditionally joyful. This joyful state should not be something we have to earn or qualify for or focus on. 'Unconditionally joyful state' is our default state. This sounds like a revelation, but it is our default state. Please remind yourselves, you need no reason to be happy, and that you are unconditionally joyful.

Buddhists have an interesting way of being happy. There is a four-point proverbial saying which goes as:

"Sorrow, sorrow, all is sorrow

Impermanent, impermanent, verily all is impermanent

Momentary, momentary, all is momentary

Empty, empty, all is empty"

In other words, suffering is inevitable, but it is inevitably impermanent and temporary. Aha! That means suffering is going to go away. One can choose to be happy looking forward to the momentary nature and disappearance of suffering. Finally, it says it is all empty! It is like saying 'everything is nothing'. That is a little harder to practice if I am in pain and suffering. I am not evolved enough to be detached from all the suffering and pain even though I have tried with some success. There is a description of some evolved saints in the nineteenth and twentieth century like Ramakrishna Paramahamsa and Ramana Maharshi who were very good at detaching themselves from cancer pain and choosing to not suffer.

To be in this state of bliss with no suffering, one has to have the following four-fold disciplines:

1. The knowledge that the real 'I' is the soul/Atma and not the physical body,

2. Discriminative ability to differentiate between impermanent material happiness or distress and the eternally permanent bliss,

3. Six-fold wealth of

- determination of control of your mind, intellect, and ego to be unconditionally calm irrespective of the conditions,

- the discipline of the sense organs,

- cessation of worldly desires,

- endurance and tolerance,

- firm faith in the infinite nature of the self,

- the concentration of the mind

4. Intense longing for our default divine infinite blissful nature.

This four-fold discipline is the prerequisite for unconditional happiness or infinite bliss or experiencing 'Infinity' and no suffering. (For the enthusiastic reader wanting to read more on these profound four-fold disciplines, I would refer you to *Tattva Bodha* and *Viveka Choodamani* by Adi Shankara. There are really great commentaries written in English by Swami Chinmayananda and there are excellent YouTube videos by Swami Sarvapriyananda.)

d. Path of knowledge: Healing with non-duality to experience Infinity

Like it is said that 'there is no other', one energy prevails everywhere. So, we have the power to heal others too through our consciousness and healing power. I also tried taking various healing treatments like Ayurveda, homeopathy, Reiki, and many others which helped me in different ways. These are different methods of transferring energy from universal energy.

One relevant and universal prayer is from Kathopanishad. We chanted this in Sanskrit every day in my elementary school, run by a Catholic organization. Thanks to Late Mr. Roman Serrao, the headmaster of my elementary school, The Little Flower Elementary School, Elinje, India for laying a strong foundation in my life.

May He (the Supreme Being) protect us both, teacher and taught. May He be pleased with us. May we acquire strength. May our study bring us illumination. May there be no enmity among us.

OM! PEACE! PEACE! PEACE!

Please read the next few paragraphs very slowly. If you wish, make notes and drawings. I am again coming back to this concept of non-duality. To be benefitted from this concept, you don't have to be a Hindu, Buddhist, Jain, or Sikh. You just have to believe that there is a divine being within us. You have to believe that within you is a part of the 'Eternal Divine Being', 'God', and 'Infinity'. You can call that 'Eternal Being' by whatever name you want. If God indeed is omnipotent and omniscient, He/She cannot be a unique property of any faith or location. If He can be 'He', why not 'She'? God cannot be sitting in heaven watching over us. If God is omniscient, He/She has to be everywhere, including here, within me, right now! He/She cannot be different for different faiths. The truth is one, the wise see it in different ways, so say the wise.

When we all have this eternal strength, why worry about a problem in our body? Why dare question the power of this eternal strength? If you do not want to give a name to that 'Eternal Being' or if you are an atheist, you can consider that we have eternal and infinite strength within us. When you have eternal strength, why worry? Having said that we are all duty-bound to do our duties. That is our *karma*. We have to take due diligence in taking the appropriate treatment from people with adequate knowledge and skill to give the best possibility for the body to heal. We cannot sit and pray assuming that the Lord will heal me. This might work for some very highly spiritually evolved people. But for most people, like me and most of you, you have to do what it takes to get the best results.

Adi Shankara's 'Six Verses to NirvaaNa' (*NirvaaNa Shatkam*), which was composed over 1200 years ago, is a set of six powerful verses, which help us to dive deep within the concept of non-duality. It negates all those which we are not. In these verses, every attachment—material, emotional, spiritual, or any other, every belief, every experience, sensation, bodily function, and our very existence is examined and negated. When we realize that the true 'I' is separate from my material possessions, we realize that the true 'I' am the witness to my possessions and things that I am attached to. In other words, 'I' am the 'subject' experiencing the possessions that I am attached to, the 'objects' experienced by me. When we realize that we cannot be both the subject and the object, each of these attachments—material, emotional, spiritual in our existence are "not me". When we realize that we are only the observer, and then we are motivated to refocus on the self as the observer. That 'observer' is referred to as 'That', 'One', '*Sat*', 'The Truth', 'Pranava', 'Now', 'Pure consciousness', 'Witness consciousness', 'Awareness', or 'that Being-ness'. I am the ever-pure blissful consciousness. And as Adi Shankara has taught us, this is the realization, which leads to the true feeling of Oneness with Universe, Oneness with Nature, and Oneness with God. 'Oneness with Infinity'!

'Who am I?' by Bhagavan Ramana Maharshi and 'Six Verses to *NirvaaNa*' by Adi Shankara, say that I am not the body. My application of these teachings was that my body has cancer, but my body is not me. Disown the body. Disown cancer. Disown the pain. My body has pain, but I am not the body. Hence I don't have pain. My body has cancer, my body is not me. Keep contemplating on it. This powerful knowledge helped me thrive in the most difficult situations where I knew that I am not the sufferer while my body is suffering and I am just a witness to it. Being witness to whatever is happening inside and outside and feeling non-attached to these worldly activities, including cancer in my body, is the key to gaining inner strength and becoming robust to challenge any sickness or life issue.

This can help any of you and it is not limited to any religion or faith. All religion meets at this point "I am that", the source of infinite energy, the underlying base of everything, a Seer to this scenery.

Six verses leading to Infinity:

Question from the Guru: Who are you?

Answer from Adi Shankara (This is my short summary of the answer):

'I am not the body, I am not the mind, I am not the Intellect

I am not what my sense organs feel

I am not what my motor organs do

I am the form of consciousness and bliss,

I am the eternal Shiva, I am the eternal Shiva (I am the Infinity)'

In 700 CE, a 12-year-old young boy met a monk while wandering around in southern India, in a place called Kolluru, along the west coast. The monk asked him, "Who are you?" The young boy who later became Adi Shankara replied in Sanskrit that he was the 'eternal Shiva'. This is the English translation of that poem. Most of the poem refers to 'who I am not' and as you keep on realizing 'who I am not', what is left is pure consciousness. Hence each paragraph of this compilation of these 'six verses for *NirvaaNa*' ends with 'I am the form of pure consciousness, bliss, I am the eternal Shiva ('Shiva', referring to God/Brahman/Infinity)'. This and many related teachings assume that what keeps changing and hence impermanent is unreal and what does not change is real. My body keeps changing every day as my body grows older. The cells keep getting replaced, body shape keeps changing every day. Hence he says, I am not the body.

Similarly, my mind and intellect change every day and hence are unreal, therefore I am not the mind and I am not the intellect. I am the form of consciousness, bliss, I am the eternal Shiva.

This poem is known as 'Six verses leading to *NirvaaNa*' ('*NirvaaNa Shatkam*').

The following is the literal translation of the poem:

1. I am not the mind, the intellect, the ego, or the memory,

I am not the ears, the skin, the nose, or the eyes,

I am not the space, not earth, not fire, not water nor wind,

I am the form of pure consciousness and bliss,

I am Shiva, I am Shiva

2. I am not the breath, not the five elements,

I am not the matter, not the five sheaths of consciousness

Nor am I the speech, the hands or the feet,

I am the form of pure consciousness and bliss,

I am Shiva, I am Shiva

3. There is no like or dislike for me, no greed or delusion,

I know not pride or jealousy, I have no duty,

No desire for wealth, lust, or liberation,

I am the form of pure consciousness and bliss,

I am Shiva, I am Shiva

4. No virtue or vice, no pleasure or pain,

I need no mantras, no pilgrimage, no scriptures or rituals,

I am not the experienced or the experiencer,

I am the form of pure consciousness and bliss,

I am Shiva, I am Shiva

5. I have no fear of death, no caste or creed,

I have no father, no mother, for I was never born

I am not a relative, nor a friend, nor a teacher, nor a student

I am the form of pure consciousness and bliss,

I am Shiva, I am Shiva

6. I am devoid of duality, my form is formlessness,

I exist everywhere, pervading all senses,

I am neither attached, neither free nor captive,

I am the form of pure consciousness and bliss,

I am Shiva, I am Shiva

Salutations to the Guru of the world, Adi Shankara. (As a sign of respect, he is considered 'Jagadguru' which means Guru of the world.)

This is a 'self-inquiry' based approach to experience the 'Infinity' right within you, without looking for God in temples, monasteries, churches, synagogues or mosques, or holy destinations. This is a 'self-experience' based approach to experience 'Infinity' or 'God' in this life, in this world, right now without waiting to die, without waiting to go to heaven! As you keep realizing what you are not, what is left is the unchanging, unmanifest, attribute-less, fearless, non-inferential, all-loving, self-effulgent, unconditionally loving 'you', the 'infinite truth' that transcends all sensations and attributes. That is the experience of 'Infinity'. You are that 'Infinity'.

'Who am I?': Self-inquiry to experience Infinity

In the early twentieth century, there was a saint called Ramana Maharshi in southern India near Chennai. He was considered highly evolved and spiritually enlightened. Once, when he was asked a question, 'Who Am I?' by one of his students (Sri M. Sivaprakasam Pillai), he answered it in a few words. Later this conversation was put together in a booklet in Tamil language and subsequently was translated to English as 'Who Am I?' He didn't read and become a realized person. He became enlightened and revealed what was mentioned in the scriptures. Interestingly his answers were somewhat similar to Adi Shankara's six verses for Liberation (*NirvaaNa Shatkam*) explained above.

This booklet consists of a set of questions and answers bearing on Self-enquiry. To maintain the purity, I have reproduced a few paragraphs from the source document.

A student asks the question: 'Who Am I?'

Ramana Maharshi's answer (This is my summary of the answer, I have done my best not to insert my interpretation):

'You are not the body, You are not the mind, You are not the Intellect

You are not what your sense organs feel

You are not what your motor organs do

You are what is left after self-inquiry and knowing what you are not

You are *existence-consciousness-bliss*

You Are Infinite Consciousness'

Mr. M. Sivaprakasam Pillai, during one of his visits, sought spiritual guidance from him and solicited answers to questions relating to Self-enquiry. This record was first published by Mr. Pillai in 1923, along with a couple of poems composed by himself. We find thirty questions and answers in some editions and twenty-eight in others. They clearly set forth the central teaching that the direct path to liberation is Self-enquiry. The mind consists of thoughts. The 'I' thought is the first to arise in the mind. When the inquiry 'Who am I?' is persistently pursued, all other thoughts get destroyed, and finally the 'I' thought itself vanishes leaving the supreme non-dual Self alone. The false identification of the Self with the phenomena of non-self such as the body and mind thus ends, and there is illumination. As one enquires 'Who am I?', other thoughts will arise; but as these arise, one should not yield to them by following them, on the contrary, one should ask 'To whom do they arise?' In order to do this, one has to be extremely vigilant. Through constant inquiry, one should make the mind stay in its source, without allowing it to wander away. All other disciplines such as breath-control and meditation on the forms of God should be regarded as auxiliary practices. They are useful in so far as they help the mind to become quiescent and one-pointed. For the mind that has gained skill in concentration, Self-inquiry becomes comparatively easy. It is by ceaseless inquiry that the thoughts are destroyed and the Self, realized—the plenary Reality in which there is not even the 'I' thought, the experience which is referred to as "Silence". This, in substance, is Bhagavan Sri Ramana Maharshi's teaching in Who am I?.

Who Am I? As all living beings desire to be happy always, without misery, as in the case of everyone there is observed supreme love for one's self, and as happiness alone is the cause for love, in order to gain that happiness which is one's nature and which is experienced in the state of deep sleep where there is no mind, one should know one's self. For that, the path of knowledge, the inquiry of the form "Who am I?", is the principal means. I would encourage you to read this booklet, 'Who Am I', that is available to buy or download online. I will just reproduce the first three questions and answers from the booklet 'Who am I?' for your reading.

1. Question: Who am I?

Answer: The gross body which is composed of the seven humours (body fluids, blood, muscle, fat, bone, bone marrow, reproductive liquid of men and women), I am not; the five cognitive sense organs, viz. the senses of hearing, touch, sight, taste, and smell, which apprehend their respective objects, viz. sound, touch, colour, taste, and odour, I am not; the five motor organs, viz. the organs of speech, locomotion, grasping, excretion, and procreation, which have as their respective functions speaking, moving, grasping, excreting, and procreating, I am not; the five vital airs, which perform respectively the five functions of in-breathing, exhalation, energy that digests and assimilates incoming energy, force that distributes life energy by causing it to flow radiating across the body, and 'upward moving' of energy, I am not; even the mind which thinks, I am not; the nescience too, which is endowed only with the residual impressions of objects, and in which there are no objects and no functionings, I am not.

2. Question: If I am none of these, then who am I?

Answer: After negating all of the above-mentioned as 'not this', 'not this', that Awareness, which alone remains—that I am.

3. Question: *What is the nature of Awareness?*

Answer: The nature of Awareness is existence-consciousness-bliss

Salutations to Bhagavan Ramana.

This is a 'self-experience' based approach to experience 'Infinity' or 'God' in this life, right now without waiting to die and without having to go to heaven that we don't know if it exists! We know that the 'self' exists today for us to experience and for that reason, 'self-inquiry' is something that all of us can do. If 'self-inquiry' is available to us, the result of 'self-inquiry' is knowing the self, which is also available to us in this life. That result of self-inquiry is the blissful experience of 'Infinity'. This experience is not a mystic experience. This experience is a secular experience that I am the unchanging, unmanifest, attribute-less, fearless, non-inferential, all-loving, self-effulgent, unconditionally loving 'I', the 'infinite truth' that transcends all sensations and attributes. That is the experience of 'Infinity'. You are that 'Infinity'. This is God, democratized for the commoners!

e. Buddhist approach to experience Infinity: I am the awakened (Buddha):

I learned this from one of the YouTube videos of Swami Sarvapriyananda. There is a story of Buddha that is relevant to experiencing 'Infinity'. Apparently, a man notices Buddha's footprints, wheels with 1000 spokes, and exclaims, "How amazing and astounding! These are not the footprints of a human being!"

Then Buddha left the road, sat at the root of a tree with crossed legs, his body erect, in meditation, confident, inspiring, calm, with restrained senses with total tranquility.

Amazed at him, the man asked a series of questions like, 'Are you God?', 'Are you a celestial singer?', 'Are you a celestial angel?', 'Are you a human being?' When Buddha said no to all these questions, the man asked him, 'If you are none of these, then *what* are you?'

Then Buddha says, "God, celestials and human beings are abandoned by me from the stem and the roots, hence I cannot be those. Just like how a colorful lotus, though born and raised in wet and dirty water, rises above water standing not smeared by the water and dirt, even though I am born in the world and grew up in this world, I am unattached to this world. Remember me as the 'awakened'. The literal meaning of Buddha is 'awakened'.

This is again a 'self-experience based approach to experience the 'Infinity' right within you, without looking for God in temples, monasteries, churches, synagogues or mosques, or holy destinations. This is a 'self-experience' based approach to experience 'Infinity' or 'God' in this life, right now without waiting to die! Pure Buddhists apparently do not believe in God, they believe in the 'awakened state', an experience that every person looks forward to throughout life. It takes a lot of contemplation to experience this 'awakened state', 'The Infinity', Buddha state'.

f. Yoga and meditation to experience Infinity:

The term yoga is used in different contexts. The literal meaning of the term yoga is 'union with', implying that 'living in union with divine consciousness'. In this chapter, I mainly refer to practicing eight limbs of yoga as described by Sage Patanjali as a means to experience or better still, be in 'Infinity'. Yoga is not just stretching and doing some exercise learned in the yoga studios, even though it is one of the eight limbs of yoga. These eight limbs are not mutually exclusive. These are like eight steps on the ladder of 'Infinity'. The eighth limb of yoga is called *samadhi*, which is a state of bliss. It is a state of unconditional bliss. It is a state of unconditional happiness. Advancing through these eight steps culminates in a state of unconditional bliss. According to yoga aphorism 2:2, the goal of yoga is not to achieve something that is lacking. It is the realization of something that is already present. Yoga helps us remove the obstacles that cover the experience of bliss, *samadhi*, a state of pure consciousness. It is believed that you do not achieve bliss. It is not something that is achieved. It is something that you already are in. It is something that you discover that you already are and you already were. Hence it is something that is your default state. It is something that you uncover and unveil. It is as though you always had the sweet and soft fruit in you, but it was covered by several sheaths and shells. When you learn to remove the sheaths and shells, you discover that you always had a sweet and soft fruit. The seven limbs of yoga preceding the stage of bliss are the sheaths and the shells. Another example to convince you that 'blissful state' is your default state is the example of little kids and adults. Little kids are always smiling. They smile for no reason. They smile even before we understand why they are smiling. At around six weeks babies start 'social smile' which is smiling at familiar faces. But they smile on their own even before six weeks. They only cry if there is a reason like wet diapers, pain, or hunger. In other words, they are always happy unless there is a reason to be unhappy. For some reason, adults are always looking for reasons to make themselves happy. The different limbs of yoga help us rediscover the 'bliss' that once was our default state. The eight limbs of yoga or the eight steps to the ladder of bliss are as follows.

Moral codes (*yama*): Non-violence, truthfulness, non-stealing, abstinence, non-receiving

Self-purification/rules (*niyama*): External and internal cleanliness, contentment, mortification, self-study, worship of God

Postures/exercise (*asana*): These are called yoga by many studios

Breath control (*pranayama*)

Withdrawal from sensory pleasures (*pratyahara*)

Concentration (*dharana*)

Deep Meditation (*dhyana*) and

Union with the object of meditation (*samadhi*)

Figure: Representation of eight limbs of Yoga as the means to be in 'Bliss/Infinity'

Going along these eight steps is a lifelong process. If you believe in rebirths, it could take more than one birth. The physical and mental components of these eight steps can be accomplished in one life, but the seventh and eighth steps are experiential and could take more evolution. Steps one to six are things you do consciously and the seventh and eighth steps are things that happen unconsciously. To maintain the purity of the practice, it is recommended that you learn this from a trained person and do plenty of self-study and contemplation. Since certain parts of yoga may not satisfy the materialistic definition of scientific truth, this state of bliss may not be palatable and/or accessible to some people. Over my life as a regular human being, scientist, researcher, and physician, I have been humbled on numerous occasions to realize the limitations of science and intellect. For that reason and from my life journey, life experience, self-study, and spiritual learning, I believe in yoga as a method to access cosmic intelligence and to experience 'Infinity' within us in this life. That experience is available to you, waiting for you to try, explore, invoke and experience. Please give yourself an opportunity for this profound experience of the fearless, all compassionate, birthless, deathless, self-effulgent, and eternal ONE truth that is beyond birth, death, and time.

Chapter 2 of the Yoga Sutras describes five obstacles to the experience of bliss. Since this book is about problem-solving and getting through the obstacle of cancer, let us study these obstacles. I thank my friend and teacher, Dr. Sriram Sarvotham for giving me clarity on these obstacles.

FIVE OBSTACLES IN LIFE ARE:

1. Ignorance

2. Ego

3. Attachment

4. Aversion

5. Clinging to life

Ignorance: This refers to the ignorance of awareness of the truth, truth of the 'Self'. The truth of the self refers to the eternal truth that the 'Self' is not the flesh and blood of the body. The true self is not the body that is affected by cancer! It is not the mind that thinks that the body is the self, that the mind is controlling, it is also not the intellect, it is the pure consciousness that is over and above the body, mind, and intellect. The true self is the 'Infinity'.

Ego: Ego gives us the labels, the adjectives that tag us to a certain gender, ethnicity, race, skin color, education, occupations, faith, country of origin, income category, type of dress we wear, type of car we drive, size of the house we live in, people we associate with. When we slowly peel off these tags and identities we refer to a person by, we lose our limited identity and we realize that we are all human beings. If we go beyond our identity as human beings, we realize that we are just living beings. If we remove that identity that we are living beings, we realize that we are a portion of the infinite world. If we go further ahead we realize that we are the 'Infinity'.

Attachment: This is the third obstacle to the realization of the self. This could be about the desire to possess something. It is about a desire to possess wealth, a desire to possess a status, a desire to possess certain goals, and certain outcomes in life. I have grown in life from difficulty having minimum means in life in India, becoming a physician in India, and now comfortably living in the US. I cannot say that I was unhappy because of a lack of funds during my childhood. I had a happy childhood and happy adult life and I am still happy now. Desires give more desires which in turn give more desires. I have grown from being attached to a comfortable life with no pain and discomfort. I have grown from being attached to a perfectly healthy life. I have grown from expecting a 'perfect problem-free life' to being happy in the middle of problems. Looking back into my life, I probably was capable of detachment even before I ever knew about my cancer. I could study medical books inside the chaotic, noisy, and crowded trains in Mumbai. In chapter 2: 62,63, The Holy Gita says that attachment to the objects of senses leads to desire, desire leads to anger, anger leads to clouding of judgment, which results in bewilderment of memory. The bewilderment of memory leads to the destruction of intellect which ruins the individual. As we detach ourselves from desires we discover the happy self that already was in us and we experience 'The Infinity' in us.

Aversion: Aversion is dislike towards something. Often we identify ourselves with our dislikes. We may dislike certain kinds of people, we may dislike certain ways of worshipping, we may dislike certain kinds of food, we may dislike certain colors, certain music, certain topics, certain political parties or certain politicians, etc. I certainly dislike cancer, pain, the discomfort of ileostomy or colostomy bags, inconvenience of incontinent life. If we commit to going beyond these dualities of likes and dislikes, we realize harmony, we realize universal love, we realize universal divinity, we realize ONEness, we realize and experience the 'Infinity'.

Clinging to life: Clinging to life comes from fear of death. This comes from the incorrect identification with the temporary body as the real self. As we practice the do's and don'ts of life, withdraw from the finite things in life, practice meditation to experience the divinity within us, we will learn to detach ourselves from our mortal, temporary body and will experience our default state, the 'Infinity'.

g. 'IK ONKAR' and 'OM': Understand this great mantra and chant to Infinity

'Ik Onkar' is called the root mantra for the people from the Sikh faith. It is also chanted by people from other faiths. The meaning of this mantra is very profound and it goes in line with the meaning of OM described in other scriptures. It is almost similar to what is described as the 'fourth state (*turiya*)' which is a state beyond the finite states of the self in the wake, dream, and sleep states (*Mandukya Upanishad*, verse 7). I have explained this in little more detail in the section on meditation under the 'Prevention' section and also at the beginning of this chapter under the section of the definition of 'Infinity'. Apparently, this root mantra is mentioned 100 times in the holy book of Sikhs, '*Guru Granth Saheb*'. I have not studied 'Guru Granth Sahib' enough to claim expertise, but I have read about it from different sources and chanted 'Ik Onkar' enough times to briefly explain this here as a way to experience 'Infinity'. I have studied the book on 'Ik Onkar', written by Swami Swaroopananda, the current head of Chinmaya Mission. Please correct me and pardon me if I make any mistakes. This is the verbal transliteration of the root mantra. I have added a few additional words to explain and understand better. But please know that 'Ik Onkar' is beyond my finite capacity to explain. It is 'Infinity'.

God is ONE, one without a second, the essence of the universe, the originator of the Universe, accessible to the entire universe

- Name is true (Truth, the absolute Truth)

- The creator

- One without fear

- One without enemy (meaning all-loving, all-compassionate)

- Beyond time: beyond death and birth

- Self-effulgent

- Blessing from the Guru as his grace

- Chant (Meditate)

- The truth today

- The truth for the eternal future

- Also the truth

Guru (Nanak) says it is truth. This was the first verse ('sound') the Guru of the Sikhs (Guru Nanak) spoke when he was enlightened. If you keep on chanting and studying 'Ik Onkar', you would advance to experiencing 'Infinity' within yourself in this life. Like I said many times in this book, experiencing 'Infinity' is available to you in this life. It does not have to be a post mortem experience. You are that 'Unmanifest Transcendent One.' You are the universal, transcendent and transpersonal existence.

Figure: OM to experience Infinity

As mentioned earlier in the book, according to *Mandukya Upanishad* and *Ashtavakra Gita*, OM is beyond cognition and absence of cognition. It cannot be sensed by the senses, it is not known by comparison, deductive reasoning, or inference; it is indescribable, incomprehensible, and unthinkable. It is pure consciousness, the pure self that witnesses the self in the wake, dream, and sleep states. It is serene, tranquil, and blissful. It is the ONE, one without a second. It makes us realize that material life is an illusion and temporary. It transcends time, space, and object. This is the real or true Self that is to be realized.

For regular people who want to try this, I would recommend you to sit upright cross-legged, with one of your heels gently touching part of your perineum (the part behind your genitals). Be in a quiet room, with lights off, with no ambient sound (switch off radio, TV, and phone), wearing comfortable loose clothes. Chant Om 21 times every day at the same time. Do this for at least a month or more at a stretch and continue forever if you like the experience.

"Om is the 'symphony of silence." —*Swami Bodhananda*

'Om is the sleepless sleep.' —*Prakash Keshaviah Ph.D. who quotes Swami Rama*

h. Universal ways to dissolve into Infinity

(Reference: *Ashtavakra Gita*, many authors have written commentaries on this, but my source is the YouTube videos by Swami Sarvapriyananda and the book on its commentary by Swami Chinmayananda.)

The book, *Ashtavakra Gita*, in chapter 1:12, says that "you are the self, you are the witness consciousness without attachment, you are all-pervading, you are complete, you are ONE, free, consciousness, inactive, unattached, desireless, peaceful, even when it revolves as 'illusion' in the cycle of births and deaths".

There is some profound and simple explanation describing four ways of dissolving the ego and experiencing the 'Self' as 'Infinity' or 'Pure Consciousness' in the fifth chapter of this very profound scriptural book on non-duality. It describes four ways to dissolve the ego explained by a sage, Ashtavakra to a knowledgeable and noble king called Janaka over 6000 years ago. I would encourage the serious learner to read the above commentary and find an expert to explain. But few points from this book are worth mentioning with reference to experiencing the Infinity' in this life before death as an antemortem experience without having to die and go to heaven.

1. **Unattachment**: You, the 'Pure Self', are the 'Truth' and are unattached to the body and the mind. Knowing that you are the pure Self and unattached, what is there to renounce? Knowing that you are unattached to the body and mind, dissolve into 'Infinity'. Remain in this undisturbed 'Infinity' and such an individual will never have to suffer misery or pain. One who remains unattached under all conditions, and is neither delighted by good fortune nor dejected by tribulation, will always be in joy. Knowing that you are unattached under all conditions, you 'dissolve into Infinity'.

2. **ONEness**: The universe arises from you like bubbles from the sea. Know that the bubbles, waves, and the sea are all ONE—water. Know yourself as ONE, one without a second. Knowing that you are the 'non-dual self', dissolve into Infinity. Knowing that you are an infinite ocean of consciousness, dissolve into Infinity. Knowing that we are all one universe with infinite love, dissolve into Infinity. Knowing that you are eternal ONE consciousness, merge into Infinity.

Recognizing this Infinity in you and you as this Infinity, dissolve into Infinity.

This ONEness has been expounded by Adi Shankara, Chaitanya Maha Prabhu, Sant Tulsi Das, Kabir Das, Meerabai, Sikh Gurus, Dalai Lama, Sai Baba, Swami Chinmayananda, Jesus Christ, and many other noble souls. This experience of ONEness can take a long time, little by little. God Krishna says in the Bhagavad Gita (6:25), "Little by little, let him attain quietude by intellect held in firmness; having established the mind in the Self, let him not think of anything". Knowing that ONEness, you 'dissolve into Infinity'.

3. **Borrowed existence of the body and mind**: The universe that you see and feel is ever-changing. My body was younger yesterday, a little older today, still older tomorrow, much older a few years later, it is ever-changing. My body or mind is never the same. It borrows existence from the real 'Self'. The real 'Self' was the same yesterday, is the same today, and will be the same 'Self' tomorrow and forever. Like a wave and the sea appear to exist in the unchanging water, the universe appears to exist in the unchanging Self, but that existence of the changing universe is 'borrowed existence' and hence is an appearance, somewhat unreal compared to the unchanging, permanent Self. This universe is the reflection of that infinite Self. Knowing that our body, including cancer, is in a borrowed existence, you 'Dissolve into Infinity'.

4. **Equanimity of mind**: This is the consequence of the above three steps. You are perfect and changeless in pain and pleasure, in hope and disappointment, and in life and death. Knowing this, be serene in pain and pleasure, be serene in illness and wellness, be serene in hope and despair, and be serene in death and life. In this state of equanimity and serenity, you 'Dissolve into Infinity'

Chapter Thirteen

Is It Possible to Experience Infinity in This Life? Is Infinity Relevant in Cancer Care?

The answer to the first question is a resounding 'yes'. The beauty of the non-dualistic Infinity is 'you are that'. The real 'you' is the 'Infinity' and all you are experiencing is what you are. Of course, it takes the knowledge of who you are and the discriminative capacity to differentiate the finite you and the infinite you. It takes sincere effort, trust, and an intense longing to experience the Infinity.

The next question is if it is possible to experience Infinity in the middle of a crisis such as cancer. The answer is another resounding yes. Know that the greatest wisdom of the Gita was taught in the middle of the war, Mahabharata. The Holy Bible was revealed after crucifying Jesus Christ for three days. The greatest of the speeches were delivered in front of massive audiences. The greatest of the sports records were broken in front of the largest audience. Michael Jordan gave one of his greatest performances when he was suffering from influenza and the whole world was watching him. The best in us comes in the most challenging times. Infinity reveals itself when Infinity is the need of the hour. Similarly, you owe yourself to unveil and experience the 'Infinity' in you right when you need it and there is no better time than now, there is no better time than when you or your loved one develops cancer.

Is this relevant to cancer care? Of course, yes! Cancer care is when we need infinite effort, infinite skill, infinite knowledge, infinite strength, infinite resolve, infinite immunity, infinite experience, and infinite bliss. If you consider 'Infinity' spiritual, it is spiritual. Spirituality should not be limited to your prayer room, temple, shrine, Gurudwara, monastery, ashram, church, synagogue, or mosque. In fact, it is a waste of your time if you limit it. Practice spirituality in your secular life. That is the need of the hour. It would be very useful and very empowering to fight cancer with infinite strength. It would be perfect to keep cancer as something not part of you and fight it out. It would be perfect if I can separate the pain from myself. Experiencing Infinity has been of immense help to me in vanquishing cancer, staying away from it, and living a blissful life.

I think I have mainly followed the non-dualistic method of experiencing Infinity along with devotional and yogic methods. But I have been the beneficiary of all the paths mentioned above. Yes, it is possible to follow all these paths. Follow some or all these paths and walk your own. Make your own path that will define itself or not define itself. The path will define itself without you intending to define it. This has been a life-enhancing, empowering, healing and peaceful experience of merging into Infinity. I hope you will find a balancing approach of experiencing the divine in you to heal you, enhance you, and enlighten you. Thank you for studying my journey. I bow to the divine in you (Namaste).

I want to end with another universal prayer from *Isha Vasya Upanishad* stressing the infinitude of 'The Infinitude" here:

"Om, That is Infinity, This is Infinity, from the Infinitude comes the Infinitude. If Infinitude is taken away from Infinitude, Only Infinitude remains, Om, Peace, Peace, Peace."

SECTION 5: CONCLUSION

Chapter Fourteen

Highlights of the Book

You get one chance to make the right decision, hence do it right the very first time.

Arise, Awake, Stop not till your goal is reached.

Do your duties with all the good skills that you have and the results will follow.

Cancer management is a team sport that you have to play as though it is the last game of your life, play it like the world cup finals where you are the captain, every team player contributes in a unique way.

Teamwork refers to the knowledge, behavioral skills, and attitudes that team members use to navigate interdependent tasks. To create an effective team with the least chance of failing, one must consider the knowledge, skills, and attitude of team members.

'No wonder kids cry when the diaper is soiled', it is very uncomfortable and demeaning to have stools in the diapers. The wet diaper should be changed as soon as it is wet.

Celebrate small victories and small progress; don't over celebrate because that will make it harder to deal with the difficult moments.

Small, repetitive steps become a path, short paths become longer paths and longer paths become infinity. (This sentence came from me, but I may have been inspired by a Chinese saying, "A journey of a thousand *li* starts beneath one's feet." from *Tao Te Ching* attributed to Lao Tzu, a renowned Chinese philosopher.)

I like support, I like to be loved. However, mercy and too much sympathy are not very helpful.

Treat a person with cancer as a normal human being. Moving on as though nothing has happened to me was a good way to adjust and rehabilitate.

You only have one choice. That is the choice to get well. You don't have the choice not to get well.

Pain management is a pain for the doctors too. If you over-treat, you are wrong, if you under-treat also you are wrong.

Get the best medical care available to you in this world, get the best doctors and the best hospital as though you only have one chance to do it right.

I think being a doctor worked to my advantage. But, don't be your own doctor. It can hurt.

The nurse manager of the surgery floor at MD Anderson washed me up for almost two hours. She was my 'Florence Nightingale'. It is a shame on me, I don't remember her name. She is from Kerala. I know many nurses from Kerala prayed for me. Thank you, my angels!

MD Anderson surgical oncology nurses are the best. Nobody said, 'I am not your nurse'. Everyone helped me when I asked for help.

Pray, meditate, and unveil the 'Infinity' in you. That is very empowering, healing, and joyful.

Explore God/Infinity within you and around you. You will find God/Infinity everywhere, in this world, today, right now. It is very empowering.

There is no use of God after death. I don't know if heaven is 'up there'. There is no use of heaven or God who is 'up there' to experience after death.

Make the prayers non-transactional if you are able to. Hierarchy of needs dictate hierarchy of prayers. Sometimes, we simply cannot help, but beg God for pain relief or healing and that is alright too!

Try to prevent cancer by surrounding yourself with the healthiest five elements: healthy food, water, air, yoga, meditation, singing, dancing, prayer, sleep and good company.

According to American Institute of Cancer Research, nearly half the US cancers can be prevented by changing our everyday habits.

Colonoscopy prevents colorectal cancer. Most people have a screening colonoscopy at the age of 45 years. You may have it earlier if your doctor recommends it. After that, have it every 10 years if you did not have polyps and every one to five years if you had polyps depending upon the type of polyp.

If you are a woman, have a mammogram after the age of 40 years and have a PAP smear after the age of 20 years.

Please stay updated with the cancer screening guidelines. They keep changing depending upon the data available.

Everybody who is born has to die, some die later than others. For the one who is born, death is certain and for the one who is dead, birth is certain. Please don't try to change my faith, I will not try to change yours.

Proselytization is a multimillion industry, too big to disregard, they misrepresent Jesus Christ and Christianity, it is an abuse of the vulnerable, it is social injustice, it has no good purpose other than recruiting vulnerable people to your faith, please don't do it.

I wish hospitals prevented proselytization in their premises instead of saying that the visiting evangelists are not hospital employees.

Using a form and name to God makes it easier to worship, repeating your preferred name for God is always available to you; the opportunity to experience God with attributes is a blessing. Feel free to worship God with or without attributes depending upon how you connect to God. It is fine if you do not believe in God and see 'Infinity' in certain human beings or non-human beings.

There is God in all of us, including YOU, the reader.

Eat, love, exercise, rest, sleep, meditate and pray.

Every individual is a divine being. Know about it, explore it, experience it, and be THAT. You are Infinity.

Chapter Fifteen
FINAL WORDS

I n this book, I have covered a few important points that have worked for me. It may work for you as well. I appreciate the support from my 'infinity' team of doctors, other health care providers, family, and friends. Playing as though you are playing the final game of your life is a good practice in anything we do in life, including dealing with cancer. Remember that the first attempt is the best attempt and hence do your best to get the best care in the world the very first time. I cannot stress enough about the determination to win, keeping a positive state of mind in the team members, and strategic planning of care. I also cannot stress enough about the multidisciplinary approach to care and including the mind-body medicine approach. Hence I would suggest that we work on all the five basic elements of nature for surviving and preventing cancer. These five elements are earth (physical body), water, fire, air, and space/ether. Hence besides taking the best treatment, eat healthy food filled with fruits and vegetables, drink clean water and avoid unhealthy water (such as sodas/sugary drinks/alcohol), breathe healthy air, avoid smoking, do some breathing maneuvers, practice eight components of yoga, do some prayer, sing if you can, dance if you like and read what you like, exercise, be grateful, sleep well and be happy. I would like to quote Elizabeth Gilbert of 'Eat, Pray, Love' fame as a recipe for happiness: "Happiness is the consequence of personal effort. You fight for it, strive for it, insist upon it, and sometimes even travel around the world looking for it. You have to participate relentlessly in the manifestations of your own blessings. And once you have achieved a state of happiness, you must never become lax about maintaining it. You must make a mighty effort to keep swimming upward into that happiness forever, to stay afloat on top of it". Stay motivated. According to Zig Zigler, "People often say that motivation does not last. Well, neither does bathing, that's why we recommend it daily." Have your share of a daily dose of motivation every day, in your own way. You deserve it today and every day.

I would add, "Be thankful and see divinity in everything and everybody". Hope you will like this book and if you do, please share with someone you care. If you have any suggestions please email me so I can edit the book to create a better future edition. Please write an honest amazon review today and share with your library and friends so I can reach more people. Thank you.

Finally,

You are not the body, you are not cancer. You are not the mind, you are not suffering from cancer.

You are not the intellect. You are the pure consciousness.

You are divine; you are 'that,' you are Brahman, you are ONE, you are ALL, you are INFINITY.

Pure consciousness is Brahman. Once you realize that, you will learn that 'You are that divine reality'.

The next step is 'Atman (Self) is Brahman'; the final step is experiencing 'I am Brahman.'

These four steps are defined in four 'great sentences' mentioned in the four primary texts of the Hindu faith called Vedas. Knowing that 'I am Brahman', I dissolve into 'Infinity'. Knowing that you are not the body or cancer, dissolve any problem by unveiling Infinity in you today, right now.

Dissolve and undo cancer with all your might, prevent and derisk cancer by creating harmony with the world and dissolve into INFINITY.

References:

American Society of Clinical Oncology (ASCO). Cancer.net. *Managing the cost of cancer care: Practical guidance for patients and families.* 2015. Accessed at https://www.cancer.net/sites/cancer.net/files/cost_of_care_booklet.pdf on February 27, 2019.

Ashtavakra Gita by Swami Chinmayananda

Cancer.net. *Questions to ask about cost.* 2018. Accessed at https://www.cancer.net/navigating-cancer-care/financial-considerations/questions-ask-about-cost on February 27, 2019.

Cancer Support Community. *Managing the cost of cancer treatment.* 2019. Accessed at https://www.cancersupportcommunity.org/managing-cost-cancer-treatment on February 27, 2019.

'Drg-Drsya-Viveka: An Inquiry Into the Nature of the Seer and the Seen by Shankara (Author), Swami Nikhilananda'

HealthCare.gov. *Out-of-pocket costs.* Accessed at https://www.healthcare.gov/glossary/out-of-pocket-costs/ on February 27, 2019.

Ik Onkar by Swami Swaroopananda

Isha Vasya Upanishad by Swami Chinmayananda

Kathopanishad by Swami Chinmayananda

Enlightenment without God: Mandukya Upanishad by Swami Rama

OM, the eternal witness by Swami Rama

Sadhguru.org

Taitreya Upanishad by Swami Chinmayananda

Tattva Bodha by Swami Chinmayananda

Viveka Choodamani by Swami Chinmayananda

Who Am I? by Ramana Maharshi

Wikipedia

YouTube videos by Swami Sarvapriyananda

Youtube videos on Upanishads and Yoga Sutras by Swami Bodhananda

Books on Patanjali Yoga Sutras by Swami Satchidananda and Swami Vivekananda

Bhagavad Gita by Swami Chidbhavananda from Gita Press

Sadhaka Sanjivini by Gita Press (Swami Ramsukhdas)

Limited Glossary, most of the verses are in Sanskrit language

1. Do everything as an offering to God:

BrahmaarpaNam brahmahavir Brahmaagnau brahmaNaahutam

Brahmaivatenagantavyam Brahma karma samaadhinaa

2. Kena Upanishad: A peace mantra.

Oṃ aapyaayantu mamaangaani vaakpraaNashcakshuḥ

shrotramatho balamindriyaaNi ca sarvaaNi

sarvam brahmopaniṣhadam maa'haṃ brahma

niraakuryaam maa brahma

niraakarodaniraakaraNamastvu aniraakaraNam me astu.

tadaatmani nirate ya upanishatsu dharmaaste

mayi santu te mayi santu; Oṃ Shaantiḥ Shaantiḥ Shaantiḥ

May my limbs, speech, life force (Prana), sight, hearing, strength, and all my senses gain in vigor. All is the Brahman (Supreme Lord) of the Upanishads. May I never deny the Brahman (Supreme Lord). May the Brahman never deny me. May there be no denial of the Brahman (Supreme Lord). May there be no separation from the Brahman (Supreme Lord). May all the virtues manifest in me, who am devoted to the Atman (Higher Self). May thy manifest in me.

3. Kathopanishad and Kena Upanishad:

OM Sahana Vavatu Sahanau Bhunaktu

Saha Veeryam Karavaavahai Tejasvinau adheetamastu

Ma Vidvishaavahai OM Shaantih Shaantih Shaantih

4. Peace mantra from Isha Vasya Upanishad:

Om poornam-adah poornam-idam poorna-aat poornam-udachyate

Om poorna-asya poornam-aadaaya poornam-evaa vashishyate

Om Shaantih Shaantih Shaantih

5. Four great sentences of Hinduism:

Tat tvam Asi [You are that (divine reality)]

Prajaanam Brahma (Consciousness is Brahman)

Ayam Atma Brahma (Your soul is Brahman)

Aham Brahmaasmi (You are Brahman)

6. Buddha's principles:

Sarvam KshaNikam, Sarvam Dukham, Sarvam SvalakshaNam, Sarvam Shoonyam.

The literal meaning is: "Everything is temporary, everything is unpleasant, everything is of its own nature, everything is void."

7. Root mantra of Sikhs (Ik Onkaar):

Ik Onkaar, satnaam, kartaa poorakh, nirbhau,

Nir vair, akaal moorat, ajooni sai bhang,

Gur parsaad, Jap.

Aad sach jugaad sach,

Hai bhi sach Naanak hosi bhi sach.

Meaning of OM from Mandukya Upanishad (verse 7) (from https://www.wisdomlib.org/hinduism/book/mandukya-upanishad-karika-bhashya/d/doc143606.html)

The 'fourth state' (Turīya) is not that which is conscious of the internal (subjective) world, nor that which is conscious of the external (objective) world, nor that which is conscious of both, nor that which is a mass all sentiency, nor that which is simple consciousness, nor that which is insentient. (It is) unseen (by any sense organ), not related to anything, incomprehensible (by the mind), not inferable, unthinkable, indescribable, essentially of the nature of Consciousness constituting the Self alone, the negation of all phenomena, the peaceful, all bliss and the non-dual. This is what is known as the fourth (Turīya). This is the Ātman and it has to be realized.

8. Succinct definition of God from Taittiriya Upanishad:

Sathyam Jnaanam Anantham Brahma

"Brahman is Existence-Knowledge/Consciousness-Infinite".

9. Four-fold wealth/qualifications as the means for liberation

(Saadhana Chathushtaya Sampattih) as told by Adi Shankara:

- Discrimination – Viveka

- Dispassion – Vairaagya

- Discipline – Shamaadhi Satka sampattih (six virtues: Tranquility of mind/shama, training of the senses/dama, withdrawal/uparati, forbearance and tolerance/titiksha, faith/shraddha, focus/samaadhaana)

- Intense longing for liberation – Mumukshutvam

About the Author

Anupkumar Shetty, MD FASN CPE, is a cancer survivor, public speaker, author, educator, Certified Physician Executive, and nephrologist at Dallas Nephrology Associates and Methodist Dallas Medical Center. He studied at Kasturba Medical College, Manipal, and furthered his training at KEM Hospital Mumbai, the University of Toronto, and Henry Ford Hospital, Detroit, Michigan.

Dr. Shetty is a renowned expert in Peritoneal Dialysis, a field in which he has delivered insightful talks for the American Society of Nephrology, National Kidney Foundation, Annual Dialysis Conference, Texas Medical Association, Dallas County Medical Society, Texas Indo-American Physicians Society (TIPS-NE Chapter) and the American Academy of Yoga and Meditation. His journey as a yoga practitioner since the age of 17 years adds a unique perspective to his professional expertise.

Dr. Shetty has excelled at all levels of study and has received multiple teaching excellence awards. He was awarded the prestigious TIPS Physician of the Year award in 2018 and the Greater Dallas Asian-American Chamber of Commerce Award in Medicine and Science in 2014.

Dr. Shetty is the author of two impactful books, 'The Power of Infinity: Health, Well Being and an Anticancer Lifestyle' and 'Hinduism Simplified' (Published in English and Kannada). He has also contributed to the medical field with over 25 peer-reviewed publications. This book,

'Navigating Cancer with the Power of Infinity' is a revised edition of his earlier work, 'The Power of Infinity,' offering valuable insights into health and well-being, directing it to those affected by cancer directly or indirectly. He is looking forward to his next books on Hinduism with the meaning of OM and wisdom from the Bhagavad Gita and some medical books on Peritoneal Dialysis and Fluid and Electrolyte Disorders.

He has survived colo-rectal cancer since 2004 and likes to share his experience of navigating cancer, and suggests every commoner to seek 'Infinity' in every situation and be the 'Infinity'.

He lives in Dallas, TX, USA, with his wife, Mala, and has two grown children. Besides medicine, his interests include sports, yoga, meditation, and reading spiritual literature. He has learned a lot of life lessons playing and watching sports. He believes that our body is a mini-world consisting of the five elements, namely earth, air, water, fire, and ether, and there needs to be harmony between the external world (macrocosm) and our body (microcosm) for good health. For that reason, a healthy diet, healthy water, healthy air, a healthy mind, and healthy social connections are very important for good health.

Dr. Shetty is deeply committed to supporting and guiding those affected by cancer. He is always ready to answer questions and offer free guidance at TPOfInfinity@gmail.com and info@infinityshetty.com. Your honest review at www.amazon.com or the Amazon website of your country would mean a lot to him, as it helps to spread his message and undo and derisk cancer in more people.

www.ingramcontent.com/pod-product-compliance
Lightning Source LLC
Chambersburg PA
CBHW061003280326

41935CB00009B/812